Atlas of Thoracoscopic Lobectomy with Bronchoplasty

Jian Li • Zhiqiang Long

Atlas of Thoracoscopic Lobectomy with Bronchoplasty

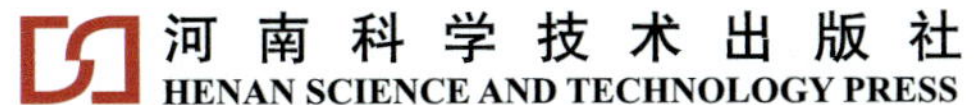

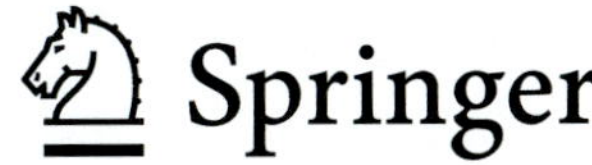

Jian Li
Department of Thoracic Surgery
Peking University First Hospital
Beijing, China

Zhiqiang Long
Department of Thoracic Surgery
Peking University First Hospital
Beijing, China

ISBN 978-981-99-5152-9 ISBN 978-981-99-5150-5 (eBook)
https://doi.org/10.1007/978-981-99-5150-5

Jointly published with Henan Science and Technology Press
The print edition is not for sale in China (Mainland). Customers from China (Mainland) please order the print book from: Henan Science and Technology Press.

This Springer imprint is published by the registered company Springer Nature Singapore Pte Ltd.
The registered company address is: 152 Beach Road, #21-01/04 Gateway East, Singapore 189721, Singapore

Reprint Preface

Atlas of Thoracoscopic Lobectomy with Bronchoplasty was printed and published in December 2014 as part of the national key book publishing plan of the 12th Five-Year Plan, and received widespread attention and praise from thoracic colleagues from the beginning. The book was nominated for the Fourth China Publishing Government Award in 2018, which gave us a great honor. At the request of readers, the book was republished in October 2019 with new content, hoping to update readers on the latest progress of surgery. However, due to space constraints, new progresses are not well interpreted.

Although the development of thoracoscopic lung cancer surgery has become increasingly mature today, people hold different insights towards the peak of the surgery. However, two standards are recognized by all: one is the radical and curative effect of the surgery; second is the least invasive approach brought by the surgery.

Colleagues had seen how lung cancer surgery could be improved with the *Atlas of Thoracoscopic Lobectomy with Bronchoplasty*, but the two-hole method was retained; Professor Li Jian's team has been trying to explore how to achieve the ultimate minimally invasive surgery. The surgical method of completing all lobectomies with a 2-cm incision emerged at the right moment. It should be said that it is a new attempt in terms of incision selection and surgical techniques.

Professor Li Jian gave a perfect interpretation of single-port thoracoscopic surgery. According to the experience of the Department of Thoracic Surgery of Peking University Hospital, most of the lobectomy specimens can be completely removed from the 2-cm hole. For the larger lobe, such as part of the upper lobe of the left lung, it needs to be removed in sections. Whether the 2-cm hole is the limit of single-port thoracoscopic lobectomy is not a bottleneck in terms of technics at present.

Up to now, the 2-cm single-port thoracoscopic lobectomy technology carried out by Professor Li Jian is becoming increasingly mature, including sleeve resection, angioplasty, and other highly difficult operations.

From the technical perspective, most operations of 2-cm single-hole thoracoscopic surgery are completed by the surgeon alone. The application of electric knife and electric hook is characteristic, and the application method is unique, which is refreshing in the aspects of exposure, hemostasis, and separation. Some special instruments, such as pen-type vascular forceps and pen-type needle holding, provide large operating space in a narrow environment. Endoscopic suture technology requires more surgical skills than ordinary thoracoscopic surgery; this book only gives a rough presentation to colleagues. Readers can also refer to the first and second editions to experience the evolution from a single operation hole of 2 cm to a single hole; the subtlety can be experienced by referring to the operation video. This book also demonstrates some cutting-edge operations, such as salvage surgery and thoracoscopic pleural pneumectomy, which are believed to bring some different feelings from others.

Beijing, China Jian Li
Beijing, China Zhiqiang Long

Contents

Part I

Basic Chapter

The technique of single-port thoracoscopic lobectomy is different from that of the porous endoscope. The operating instrument and the endoscope are displayed on the same axis, so the operation is usually performed on a single plane. Whether from top to bottom or from front to back, the operating instrument is usually operated in the same direction as the thoracoscopic endoscope. To achieve the same or even better results as open surgery, 2-cm single-hole thoracoscopic bronchoplasty lobectomy perfectly demonstrates this feature. Lobotomy is a standard and basic operation in lung cancer surgery. In this book, various radical operations for lung cancer such as the upper lobe of the left lung are shown. Electrotomy is the distinctive feature of 2-cm bronchoplasty lobectomy. The length of the disposable conventional lengthening electric knife is about 16.5 cm (as shown in the figure below). Compared with the electric hook, it is shorter and has good stability. It can reach all parts of the hilum of the lung through the incision. For example, after the bending of the electric knife head, there are some techniques, such as point, pick, hook, probe, and squeeze, which the readers can carefully experience with the operation video.

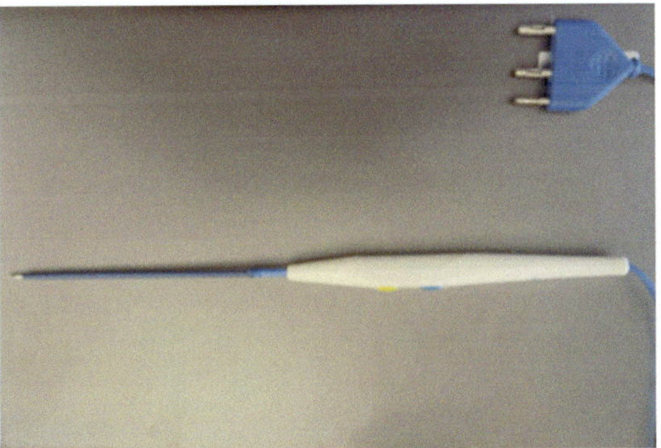

Disposable extension electric knife

1 Selection of Incision

Generally, the selection of incisions is based on the principle of fully exposing the operating field. For endoscopic surgery, the current endoscopic display system can clearly expose all directions of the operating field, and due to the development of endoscopic technology, various complex operations can be completed under the endoscope. Therefore, the location of the incision is selected mainly based on the following factors: One is to minimize the compression and compression of the intercostal nerve and tissue by the thoracoscope itself in the process of thoracoscopic surgery to prevent the occurrence of postoperative pain. Second, it is closest to the hilum of the lung, which is easier to control the hilum blood vessels, convenient to block the pulmonary blood vessels for vascular suture and forming, and avoid the conversion to thoracotomy caused by emergencies. Third, it is convenient for lymph node dissection; and finally, the size of the incision to extract the specimen. After a long period of clinical exploration, we designed an incision of about 2 cm between the third intercostal anterior axillary line and the midaxillary line as the standard incision for lobectomy of tumors less than 3 cm in diameter. This single-hole incision met all our requirements for single-hole thoracoscopic incision. Its advantage is that the laparoscope is basically parallel to the hilum of the lung, which avoids the squeezing of the intercostal nerve due to the upward exposure of the thoracoscope during the operation. However, since the intercostal nerve is located below the costal margin during the operation under the hilum of the lung, the operation of thoracoscope and instruments above the costal margin does not cause injury to the intercostal nerve. Secondly, the incision is relatively forward, basically parallel to the hilum of the lung, and can be operated in the horizontal direction, especially convenient to control the pulmonary blood vessels in the pericardium. Another advantage of these openings is the convenience of lymph node dissection in the upper mediastinum, and the shorter distance and greater operating space compared to the fourth or fifth intercostal incision. It requires a certain skill to obtain the specimen with a 2-cm incision, and it is beneficial to remove the specimen by completely eliminating pneumorrhagia.

J. Li, Z. Long, *Atlas of Thoracoscopic Lobectomy with Bronchoplasty*,
https://doi.org/10.1007/978-981-99-5150-5_1

2 Excision of the Right Superior Lobe of Lung

There are many methods for excision of the upper lobe of the right lung, including anterior approach, posterior approach, and retrograde excision. Due to the application of bronchoplasty method, the 2-cm incision is characterized by the fact that the surgical incision is parallel to the upper lobe bronchus of the right lung. Starting from the upper lobe bronchus of the right lung, the electric knife can cut off the bronchus, and the lymph nodes around the bronchus can be completely excised. After amputation, the whole upper lobe of the right lung became elastic, the length of free blood vessels increased relatively, and the anterior-posterior separation was easier. Bronchoplasty has two significant advantages in the application of lobectomy. One is that it can be removed to the maximum extent. Compared with the bronchoplasty by napping bronchial stump and ligation and suture, the length of bronchoplasty is significantly increased. Second, because no bronchial stump remains dead space, postoperative irritating cough, sputum, and other symptoms are significantly reduced. Since the incision and the superior pulmonary vein are essentially at the same level, the application of instrumentation to remove the vein requires that the artery behind it be removed. This video is about surgery in 2016. Readers can compare it with the following chapters and experience the evolution of surgical techniques (Figs. 2.1, 2.2, 2.3, 2.4, 2.5, 2.6, 2.7, 2.8, and 2.9).

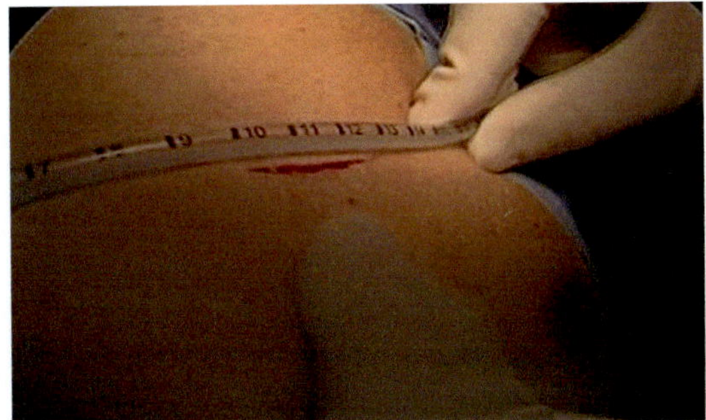

Fig. 2.1 Select the incision. The incision is 2 cm between anterior axillary line and midaxillary line in the third intercostal space

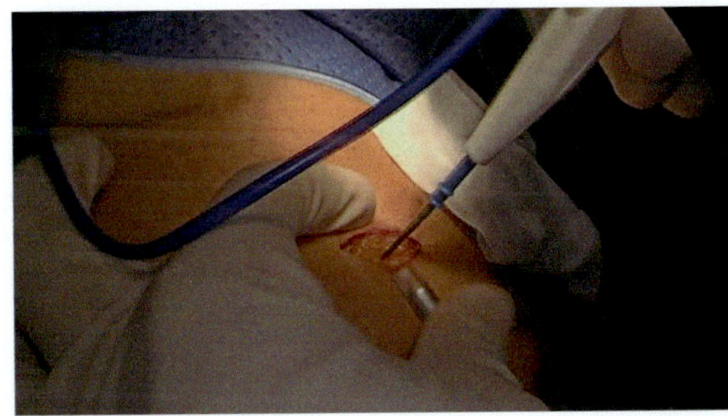

Fig. 2.2 The subcutaneous and muscular layers were incised. The subcutaneous and muscular tissues were incised layer by layer and the thoracic cavity was entered

J. Li, Z. Long, *Atlas of Thoracoscopic Lobectomy with Bronchoplasty*,
https://doi.org/10.1007/978-981-99-5150-5_2

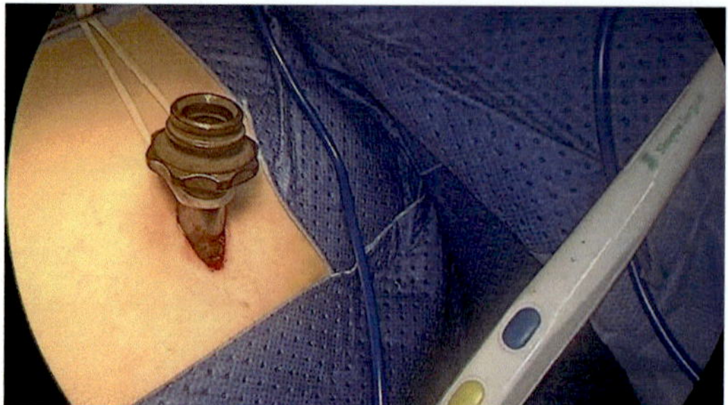

Fig. 2.3 Due to the small incision, the thoracoscope is difficult to put in, so the lumpectomy can be put in by trocar first, and then pull out the incision and leave the lumpectomy in the chest cavity

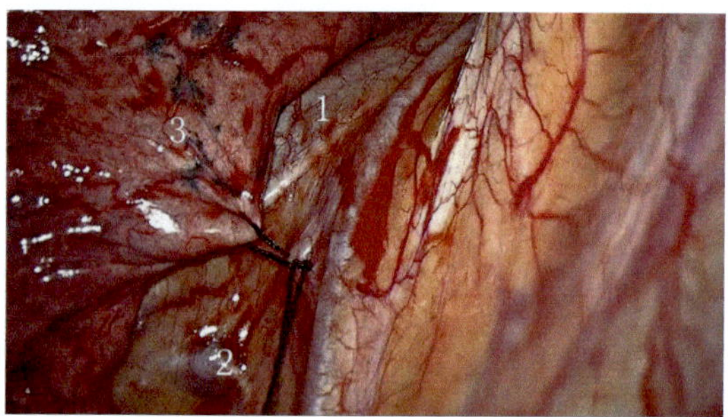

Fig. 2.4 1—Right innominate vein, 2—right internal mammary vein, 3—superior lobe of right lung. A marker suture is placed 3 cm above the pre-resected tumor tissue, which is sutured together with the chest wall to provide a pulling effect

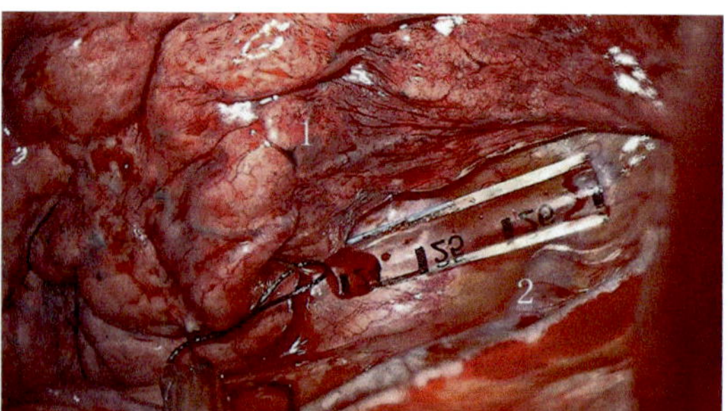

Fig. 2.5 1—Superior lobe of right lung, 2—right internal mammary vein. A marker suture is placed 3 cm below the pre-resected tumor tissue

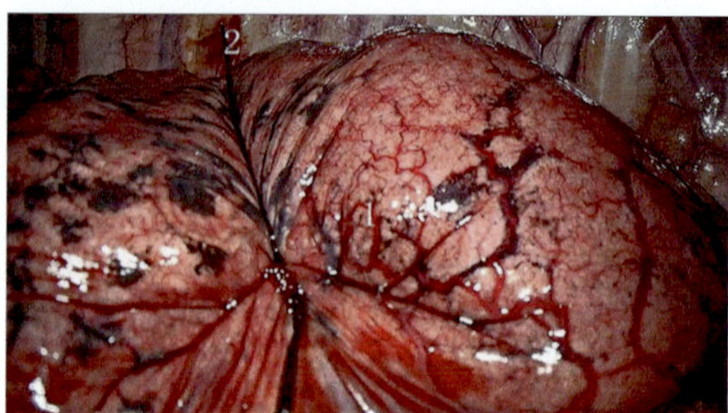

Fig. 2.6 1—Superior lobe of right lung, 2—posterior chest wall. Parallel to the front up and down marker suture, a marker suture is placed 3 cm behind the pre-resected tumor tissue and fixed to the posterior chest wall

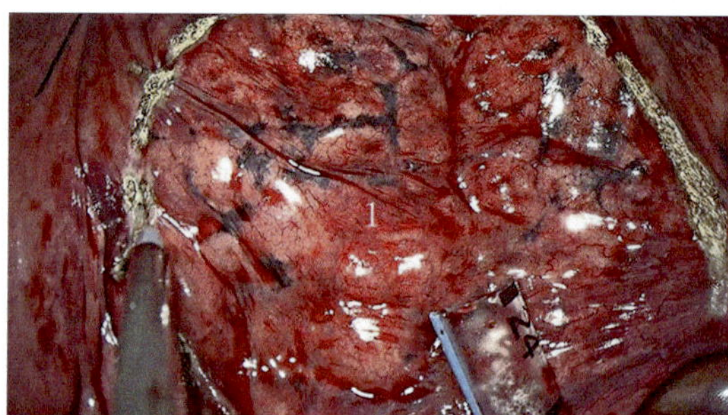

Fig. 2.7 1—Superior lobe of right lung. The extent of resection is indicated on the lung surface with an electrotome

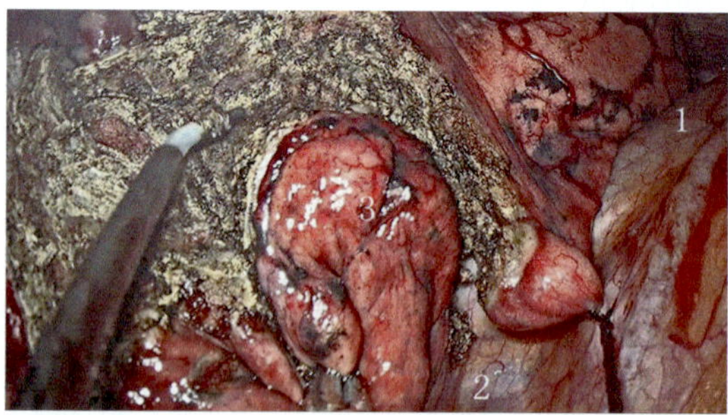

Fig. 2.8 1—Right innominate vein, 2—right internal mammary vein, 3—right innominate vein. Excise the lung tissue along the marker suture

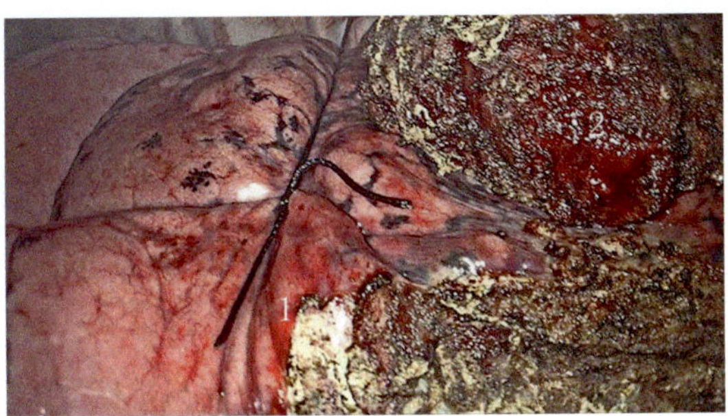

Fig. 2.9 1—Superior lobe of right lung, 2—resected lung specimen. The resected specimen is sent for rapid pathological examination, which shows an invasive adenocarcinoma, and a right upper lobectomy is performed

Surgical features: Thoracoscopic electrotome resection of pulmonary lesions requires a good spatial concept to ensure adequate incisal margin. In this case, thoracoscopic distance setting was used to determine the incisal margin, and certain tension was provided by fixing lung tissue to facilitate electrotome resection of pulmonary lesions (Figs. 2.10, 2.11, 2.12, 2.13, 2.14, 2.15, 2.16, 2.17, 2.18, 2.19, 2.20, 2.21, 2.22, 2.23, 2.24, 2.25, 2.26, 2.27, 2.28, 2.29, 2.30, 2.31, 2.32, 2.33, 2.34, 2.35, 2.36, 2.37, 2.38, 2.39, 2.40, 2.41, 2.42, 2.43, 2.44, 2.45, 2.46, and 2.47).

Surgical features: Anterior dissection of subcarinal lymph nodes is one of the advantages of the third intercostal incision. After the anterior trunk of the right superior lobar artery and the superior pulmonary vein are severed, the right main bronchi behind the pulmonary artery can be easily exposed by lifting the right superior lobar bronchi parallel to the incision. The subcarinal lymph nodes can be dissected along the lower trachea and behind the pericardium, and the dissection of the superior mediastinum can be combined with the dissection of the lymph nodes.

Summary: The difficulty of pulmonary lobectomy with a 2-cm incision lies in the intraoperative dissection of the whole lymph nodes and the removal of the specimen; this case of right upper lung lobectomy demonstrates the skill of dissection of subcarinal lymph nodes from anterior, requiring the operator to have a good spatial anatomical concept and to operate gently and accurately. The bronchoplasty performed creates the conditions for specimen removal as the bronchi are severed earlier, their intrapulmonary gases are fully expelled, and the lung is further reduced in size. This method is also used in subsequent chapters and will not be repeated.

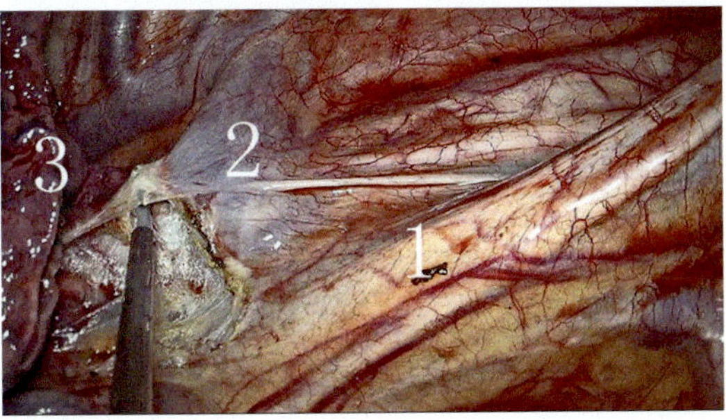

Fig. 2.10 1—Superior vena cava, 2—arch of azygos vein, 3—superior lobe of right lung. Excise the mediastinal pleura along the inferior border of arch of azygos vein

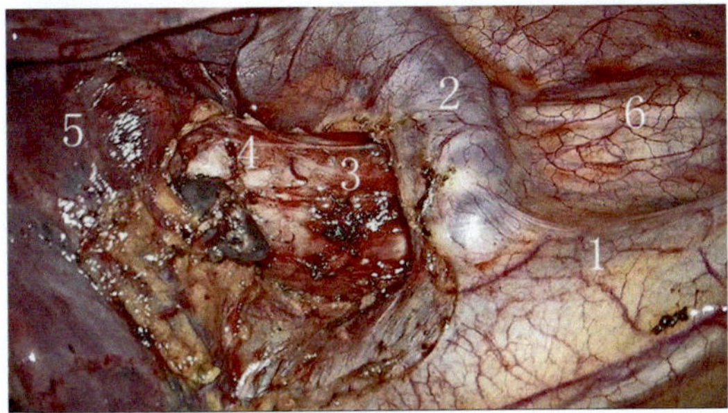

Fig. 2.11 1—Superior vena cava, 2—arch of azygos vein, 3—right principal bronchus, 4—right superior lobar bronchus, 5—superior lobe of right lung, 6—trachea. Lymphatic and adipose tissues are dissected along the right principal bronchus downward to reveal the right superior lobar bronchus

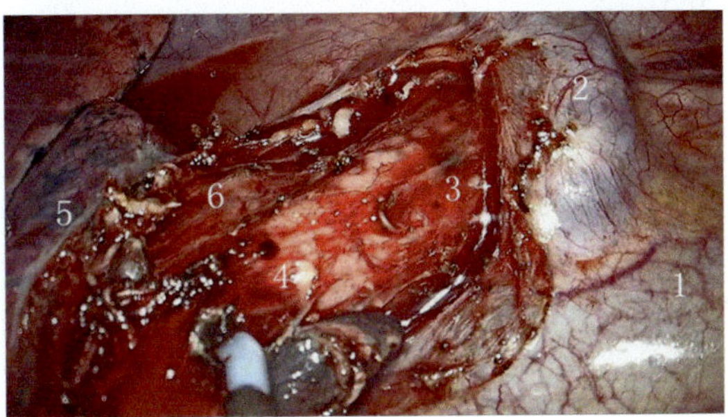

Fig. 2.12 1—Superior vena cava, 2—arch of azygos vein, 3—right principal bronchus, 4—right superior lobar bronchus, 5—superior lobe of right lung, 6—right middle segment bronchus. Dissect the lymph node along the right principal bronchus backward to reveal the right middle segment bronchus

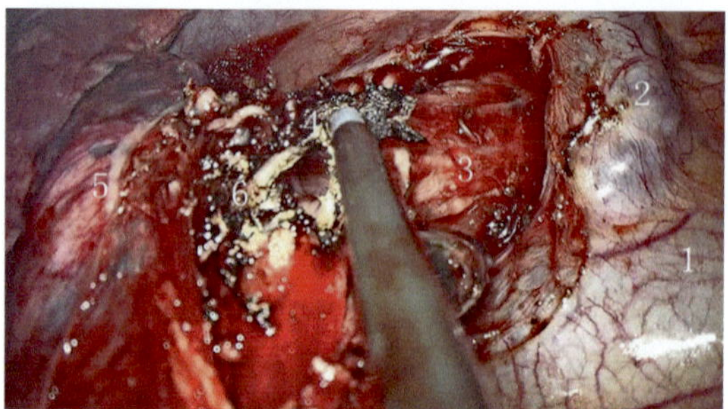

Fig. 2.13 1—Superior vena cava, 2—arch of azygos vein, 3—right principal bronchus, 4—right superior lobar bronchial stump, 5—superior lobe of right lung, 6—right middle segment bronchus. Cut off the right superior lobar bronchus at the opening of right superior lobar bronchus

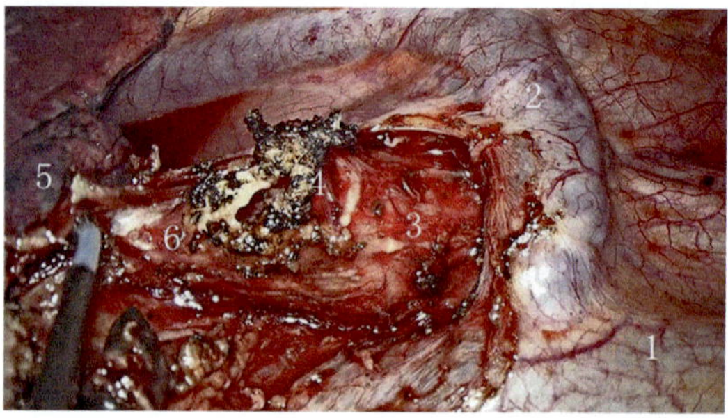

Fig. 2.14 1—Superior vena cava, 2—arch of azygos vein, 3—right principal bronchus, 4—right superior lobar bronchial stump, 5—superior lobe of right lung, 6—right middle segment bronchus. Dissect the lymph node along the right middle segment bronchus downward

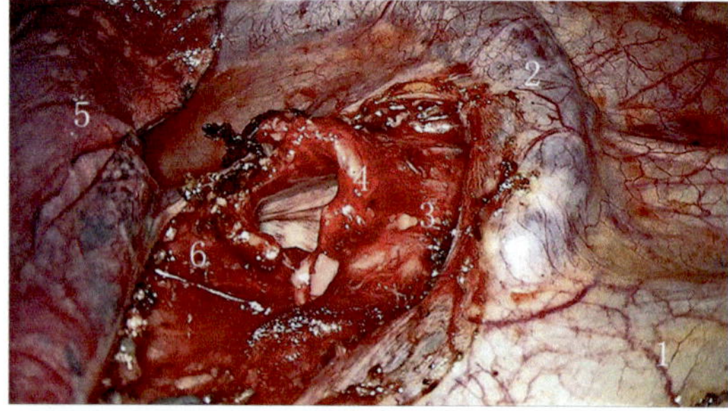

Fig. 2.15 1—Superior vena cava, 2—arch of azygos vein, 3—right principal bronchus, 4—right superior lobar bronchial stump, 5—superior lobe of right lung, 6—right middle segment bronchus. Trim the right superior lobar bronchial stump so that the cartilaginous part of the stump anteriorly becomes V-shaped to avoid angulation during suturing

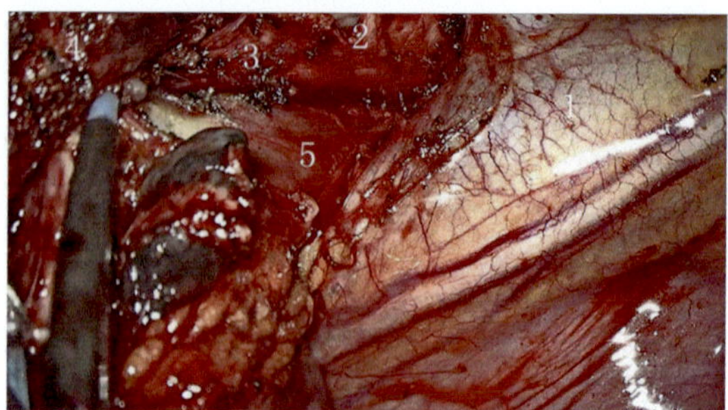

Fig. 2.16 1—Superior vena cava, 2—right superior lobar bronchial stump, 3—right middle segment bronchus, 4—superior lobe of right lung, 5—anterior trunk of right superior lobar artery. Lymphatic and adipose tissues in front of right middle segment bronchus and behind the anterior trunk of right superior lobar artery are dissected

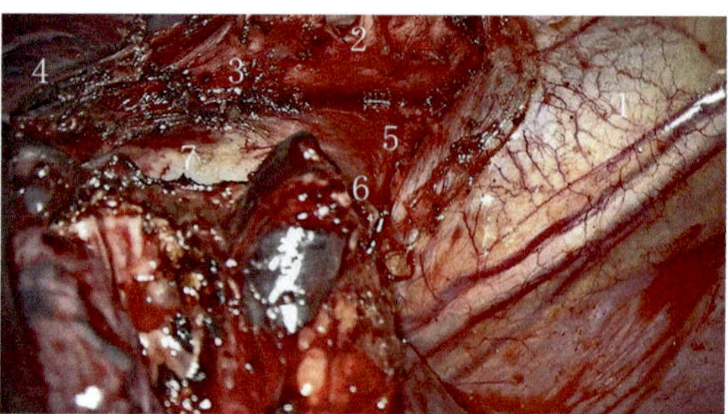

Fig. 2.17 1—Superior vena cava, 2—right superior lobar bronchial stump, 3—right middle segment bronchus, 4—inferior lobe of right lung, 5—anterior trunk of right superiorlobarartery,6—superiorlobeofrightlung,7—interlobar trunk of right pulmonary artery. Lymphatic and adipose tissues between right middle segment bronchus and the anterior trunk of right superior lobar artery are dissected

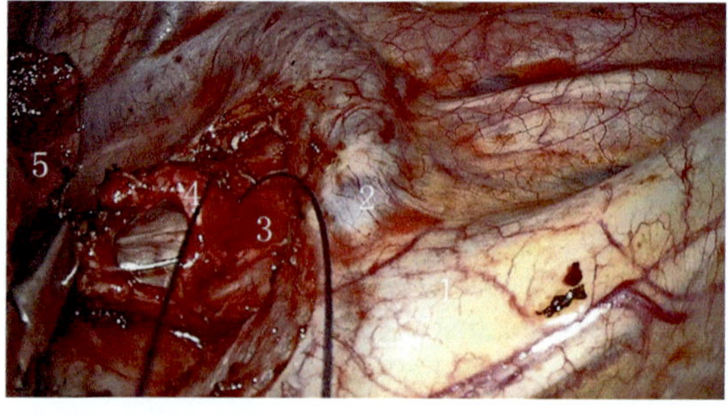

Fig. 2.18 1—Superior vena cava, 2—arch of azygos vein, 3—right principal bronchus, 4—right superior lobar bronchial stump, 5—superior lobe of right lung. Use 3-0PDSII for continuous suture of right superior lobar bronchial stump

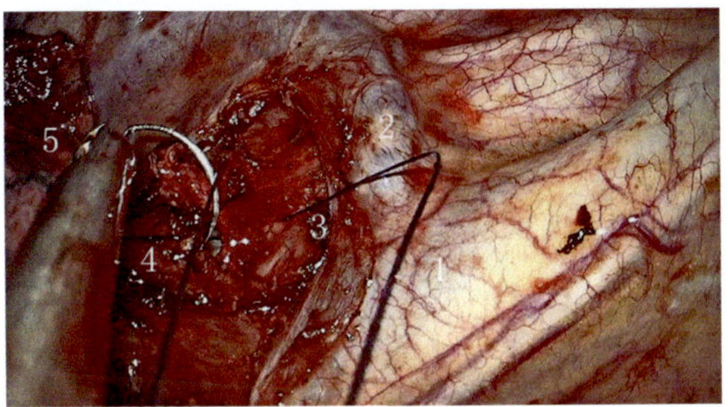

Fig. 2.19 1—Superior vena cava, 2—arch of azygos vein, 3—right principal bronchus, 4—right middle segment bronchus, 5—superior lobe of right lung. Take continuous suture of right superior lobar bronchial stump

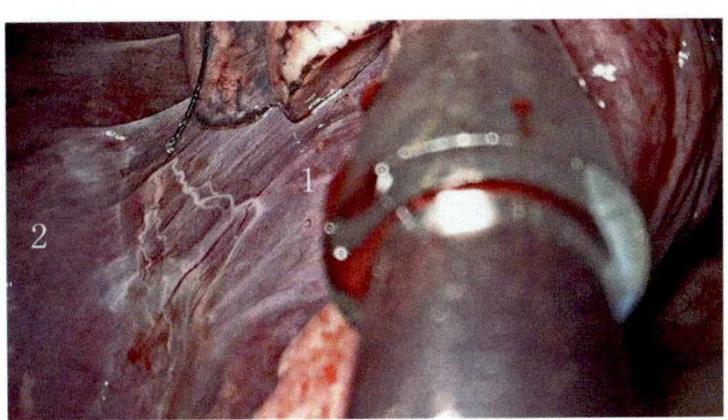

Fig. 2.22 1—Superior lobe of right lung, 2—middle lobe of right lung. Reveal horizontal fissure

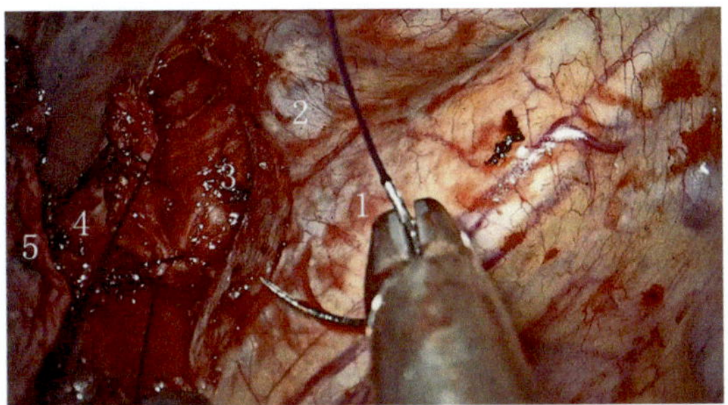

Fig. 2.20 1—Superior vena cava, 2—arch of azygos vein, 3—right principal bronchus, 4—right middle segment bronchus, 5—superior lobe of right lung. Take continuous suture of right superior lobar bronchial stump, showing the V-shaped stump of the closed anterior bronchus

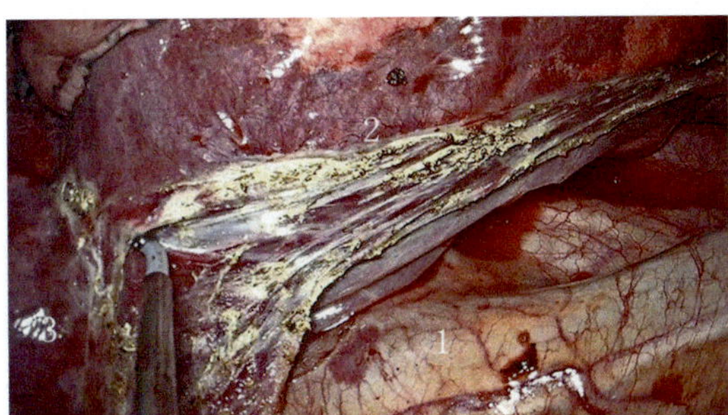

Fig. 2.23 Cut the horizontal fissure. 1—Superior vena cava, 2—superior lobe of right lung, 3—inferior lobe of right lung. Cut the horizontal fissure from anterior to posterior

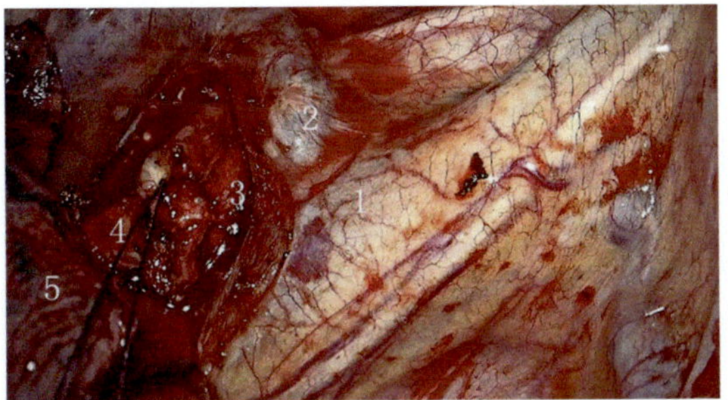

Fig. 2.21 1—Superior vena cava, 2—arch of azygos vein, 3—right principal bronchus, 4—right middle segment bronchus, 5— superior lobe of right lung. Suture of right superior lobar bronchial stump is finished

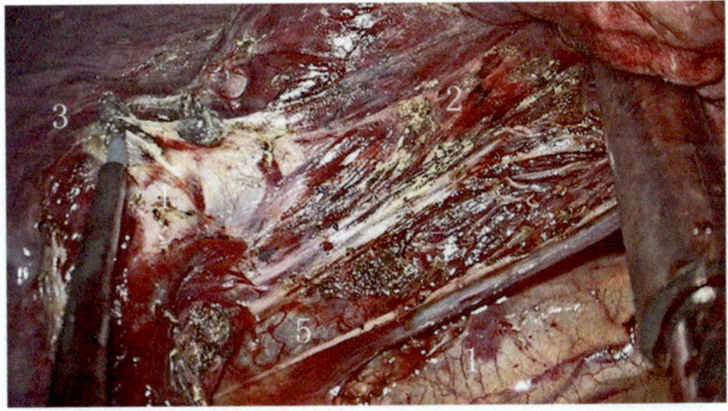

Fig. 2.24 1—Superior vena cava, 2—superior lobe of right lung, 3—middle lobe of right lung, 4—right middle pulmonary artery, 5—right superior pulmonary vein. Interlobar lymphatic and adipose tissues are dissected along the right middle pulmonary artery upward

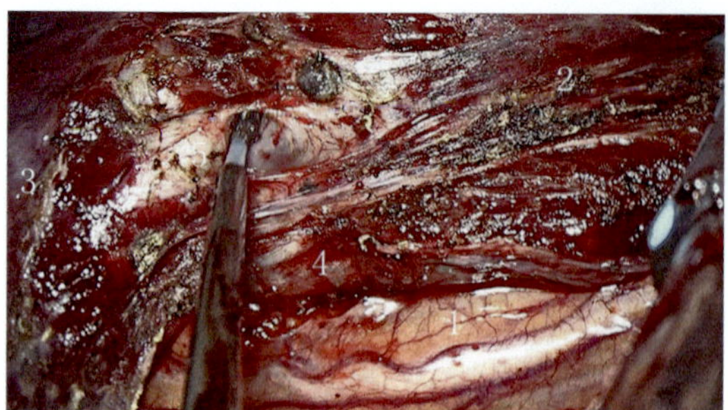

Fig. 2.25 1—Superior vena cava, 2—superior lobe of right lung, 3—middle lobe of right lung, 4—right superior pulmonary vein, 5—right middle pulmonary artery. Interlobar lymphatic and adipose tissues are dissected along middle lobe of right lung backward

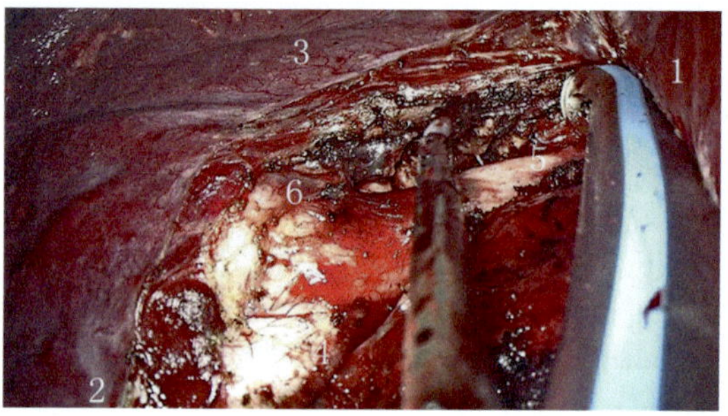

Fig. 2.26 1—Superior lobe of right lung, 2—middle lobe of right lung, 3—inferior lobe of right lung, 4—right middle pulmonary artery, 5—right superior pulmonary artery, 6—right inferior pulmonary artery. Continue to dissect the lymph node backward to reveal the beginning of right inferior pulmonary artery, and connect to the lymph node of right middle segment bronchus dissected backward

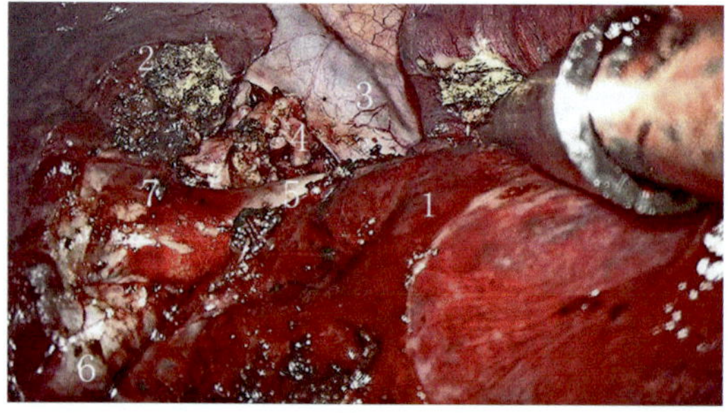

Fig. 2.27 1—Superior lobe of right lung, 2—inferior lobe of right lung, 3—arch of azygos vein, 4—right superior lobar bronchial stump, 5—posterior segment artery of superior lobe of right lung, 6—right middle pulmonary artery, 7—right inferior pulmonary artery. Cut the oblique fissure backward, and dissect the lymphatic and adipose tissues upward

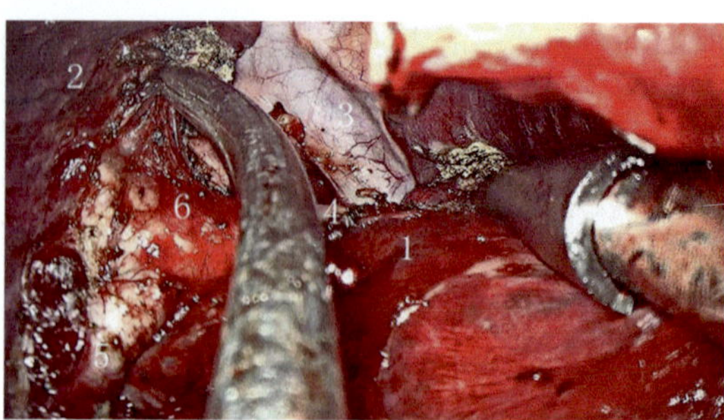

Fig. 2.28 1—Superior lobe of right lung, 2—inferior lobe of right lung, 3—arch of azygos vein, 4—posterior segment artery of superior lobe of right lung, 5—right middle pulmonary artery, 6—right inferior pulmonary artery. Dissect the lymph node beside the right middle pulmonary artery

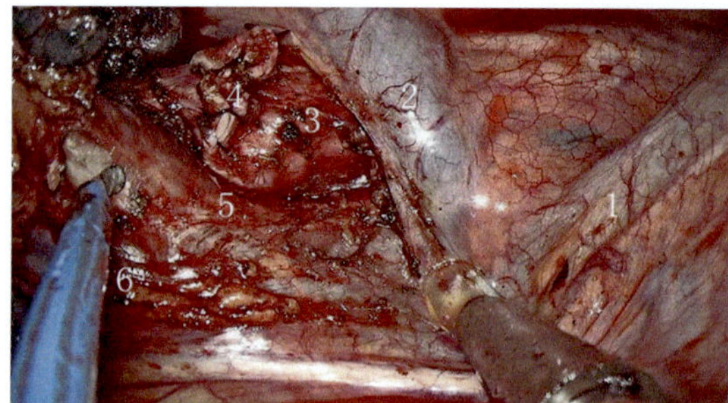

Fig. 2.29 1—Superior vena cava, 2—arch of azygos vein, 3—right principal bronchus, 4—right superior lobar bronchial stump, 5—anterior trunk of right superior lobar artery, 6—right superior pulmonary vein. Pull the superior lobe of right lung downward, open the vascular sheath of the right superior lobar artery, and dissect the lymphatic and adipose tissues downward

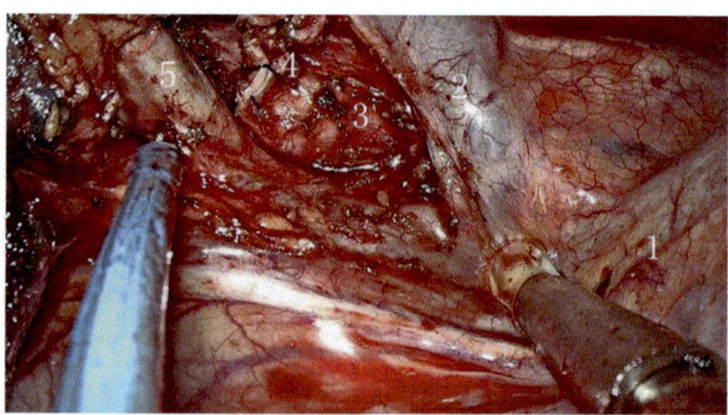

Fig. 2.30 1—Superior vena cava, 2—arch of azygos vein, 3—right principal bronchus, 4—right superior lobar bronchial stump, 5—anterior trunk of right superior lobar artery. Dissect the lymphatic and adipose tissues in front of right superior lobar artery and behind the right superior pulmonary vein downward

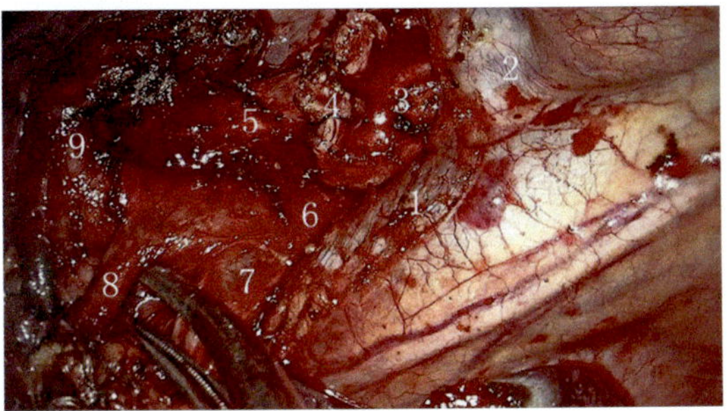

Fig. 2.31 1—Superior vena cava, 2—arch of azygos vein, 3—right principal bronchus, 4—right superior lobar bronchial stump, 5—right middle segment bronchus, 6—right pulmonary trunk, 7—anterior trunk of right superior lobar artery, 8—posterior segment artery of superior lobe of right lung, 9—inferior lobe of right lung. Dissect the lymph node along the posterior pulmonary artery downward to reveal the posterior segment artery of superior lobe of right lung

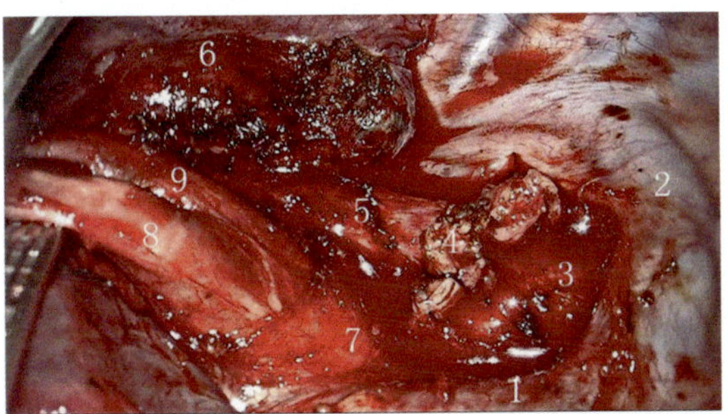

Fig. 2.32 1—Superior vena cava, 2—arch of azygos vein, 3—right principal bronchus, 4—right superior lobar bronchial stump, 5—right middle segment bronchus, 6—inferior lobe of right lung, 7—right pulmonary trunk, 8—anterior trunk of right superior lobar artery, 9—posterior segment artery of superior lobe of right lung. Cut off the anterior trunk of right superior lobar artery and posterior segment artery of superior lobe of right lung with Endo-GIA Stapler

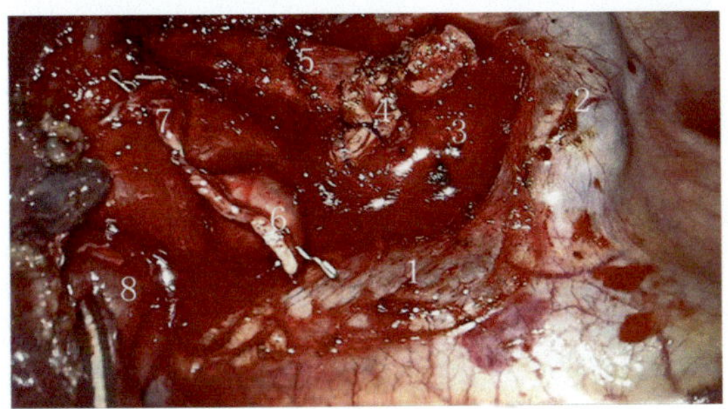

Fig. 2.33 1—Superior vena cava, 2—arch of azygos vein, 3—right principal bronchus, 4—right superior lobar bronchial stump, 5—right middle segment bronchus, 6—anterior trunk of right superior lobar artery, 7—posterior segment artery of superior lobe of right lung, 8—right superior pulmonary vein. Dissect the lymph node along the upper right superior pulmonary vein downward

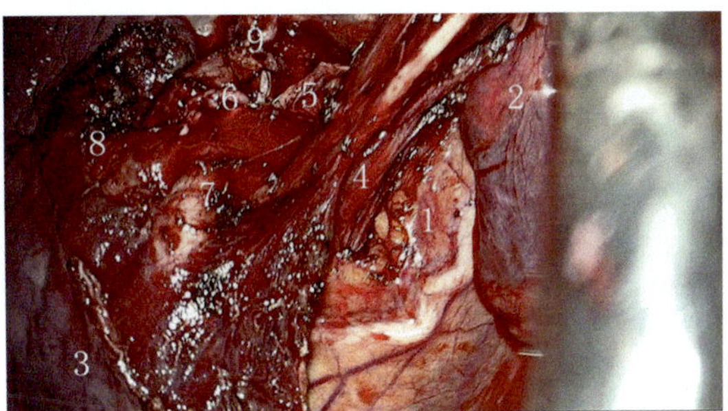

Fig. 2.34 1—Superior vena cava, 2—superior lobe of right lung, 3—middle lobe of right lung, 4—right superior pulmonary vein, 5—anterior trunk of right superior lobar artery stump, 6—posterior segment artery stump of superior lobe of right lung, 7—right middle pulmonary artery, 8—inferior lobe of right lung, 9—posterior segment artery of superior lobe of right lung. Reveal the right superior pulmonary vein completely

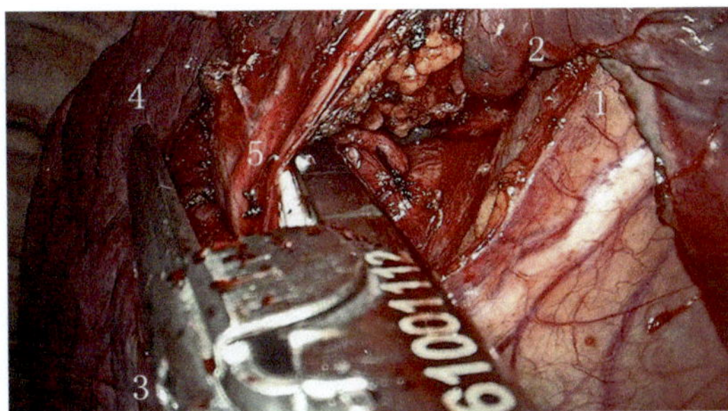

Fig. 2.35 1—Superior vena cava, 2—superior lobe of right lung, 3—middle lobe of right lung, 4—inferior lobe of right lung, 5—right superior pulmonary vein. Interrupt the right superior pulmonary vein with Endo-GIA Stapler

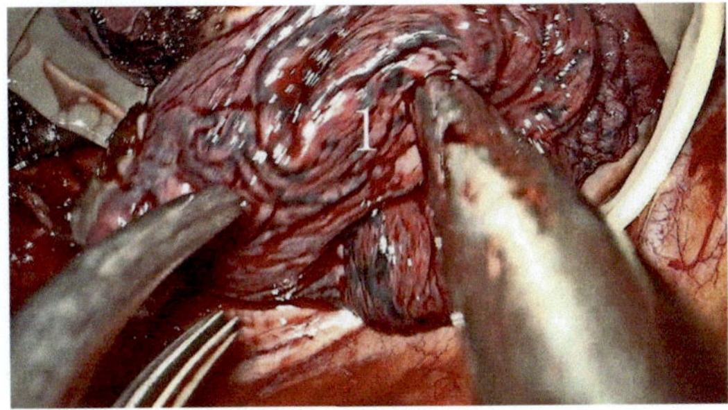

Fig. 2.36 1—Resected specimen of superior lobe of right lung. Superior lobe of right lung is put into the glove and taken out

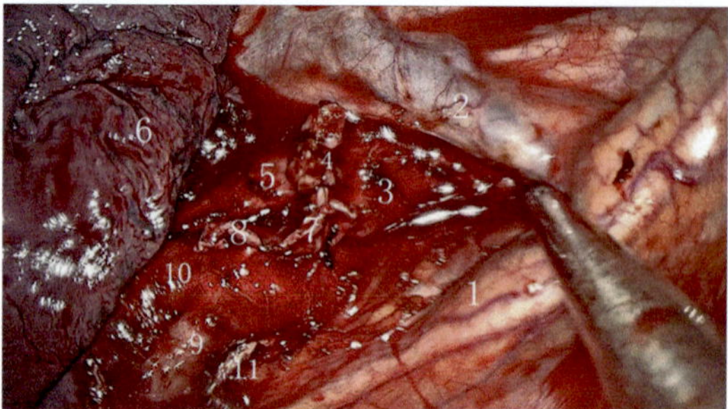

Fig. 2.37 1—Superior vena cava, 2—arch of azygos vein, 3—right principal bronchus, 4—right superior lobar bronchial stump, 5—right middle segment bronchus, 6—inferior lobe of right lung, 7—anterior trunk of right superior lobar artery, 8—posterior segment artery of superior lobe of right lung, 9—right middle pulmonary artery, 10—right inferior pulmonary artery, 11—right superior pulmonary vein. After resection of superior lobe of right lung

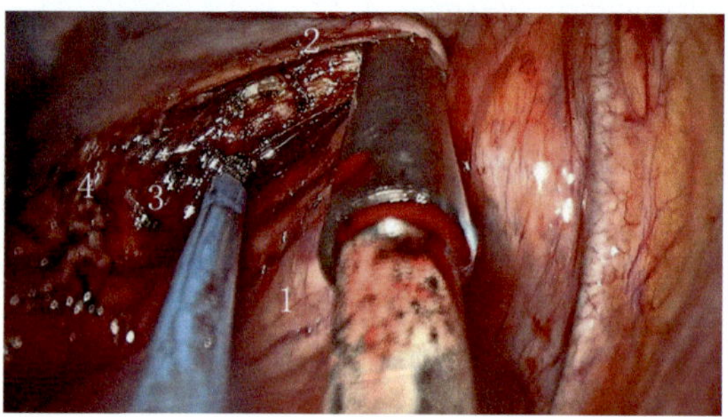

Fig. 2.38 1—Superior vena cava, 2—arch of azygos vein, 3—right principal bronchus, 4—right superior lobar bronchial stump. Pull up the arch of azygos vein and dissect the lymph node along the right principal bronchus upward

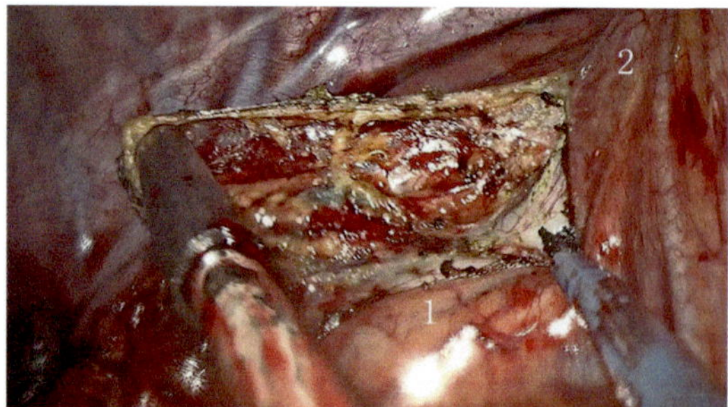

Fig. 2.39 1—Superior vena cava, 2—right innominate vein. Open the superior mediastinum pleura and dissect the lymph node along the surface of superior vena cava

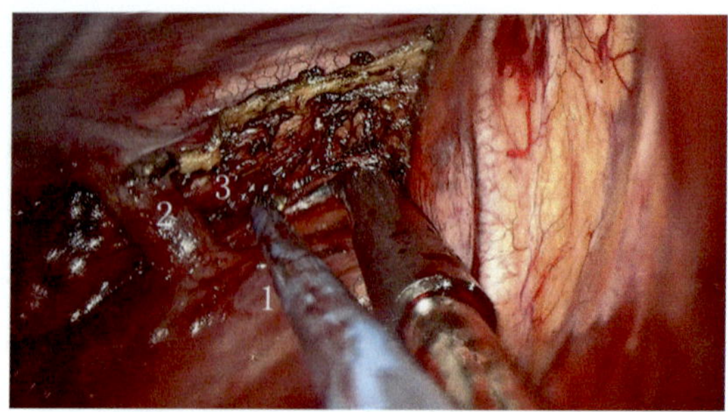

Fig. 2.40 1—Superior vena cava, 2—arch of azygos vein, 3—trachea. Dissect the lymph node along the anterior trachea upward

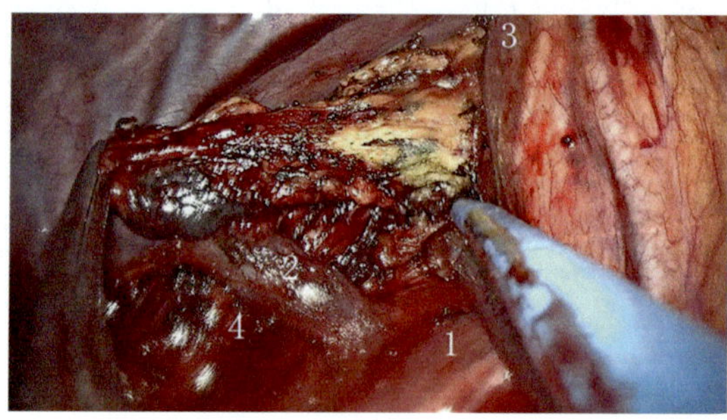

Fig. 2.41 1—Superior vena cava, 2—arch of azygos vein, 3—right innominate vein, 4—right principal bronchus. Lymphatic and adipose tissues below the right innominate vein are dissected

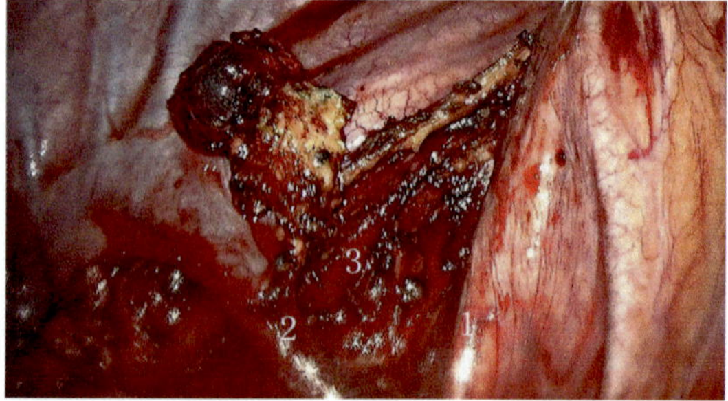

Fig. 2.42 1—Superior vena cava, 2—arch of azygos vein, 3—trachea. After the upper mediastinal lymph node system dissection

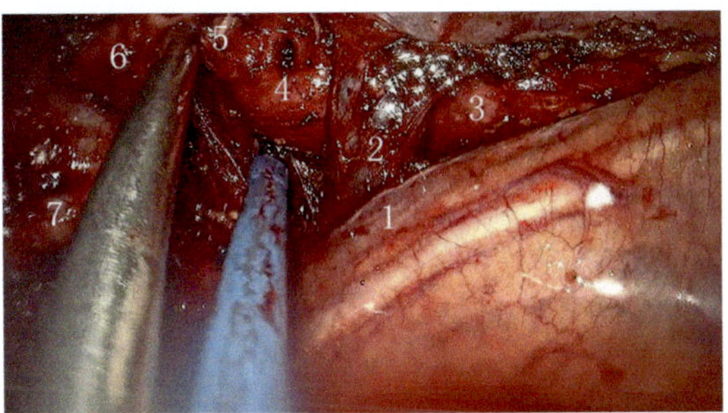

Fig. 2.43 1—Superior vena cava, 2—arch of azygos vein, 3—trachea, 4—right principal bronchus, 5—right superior lobar bronchial stump, 6—right middle segment bronchus, 7—right middle pulmonary artery. Pull up the right middle segment bronchus and dissect the lymph node along the right principal bronchus downward

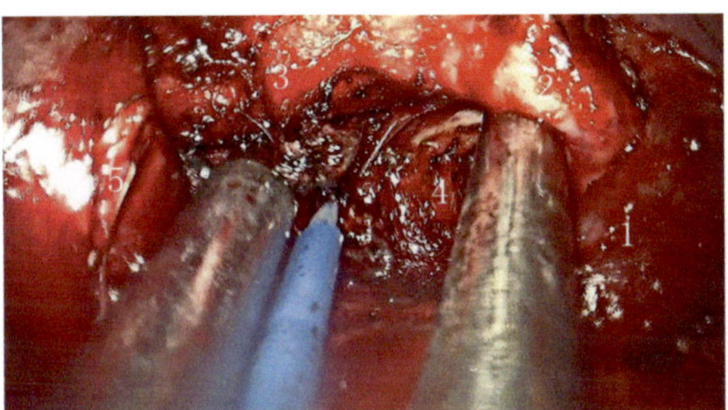

Fig. 2.44 1—Arch of azygos vein, 2—right principal bronchus, 3—right middle segment bronchus, 4—left principal bronchus, 5—posterior segment artery of superior lobe of right lung. Dissect the lymph node along the right principal bronchus backward and reveal the principal bronchus

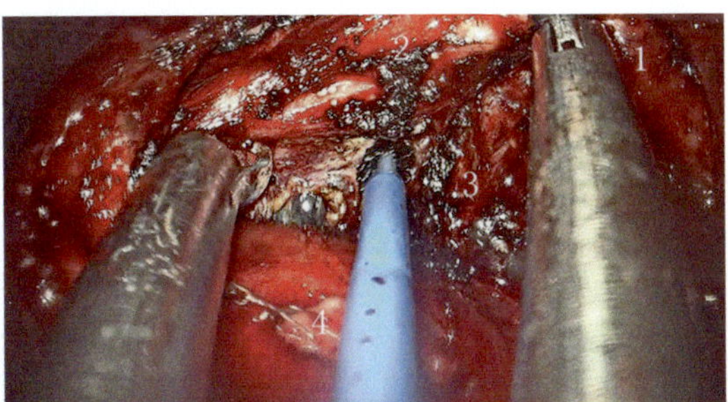

Fig. 2.45 1—Right principal bronchus, 2—right middle segment bronchus, 3—left principal bronchus, 4—anterior trunk of right superior lobar artery. Dissect the lymph node along the right middle segment bronchus backward and downward

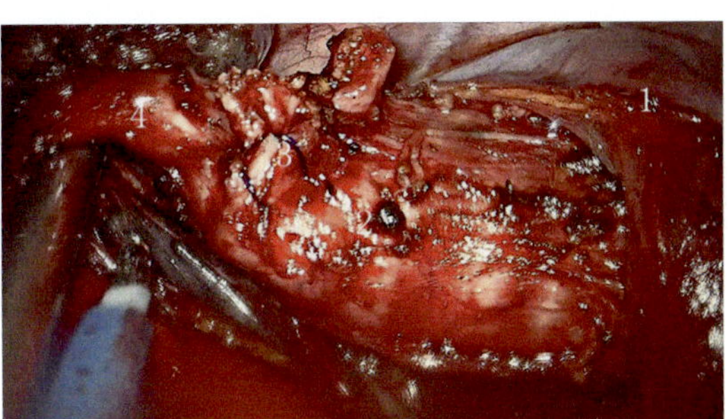

Fig. 2.46 1—Arch of azygos vein, 2—right principal bronchus, 3—right superior lobar bronchial stump, 4—right middle segment bronchus. Resect the infracarinal lymph node en bloc

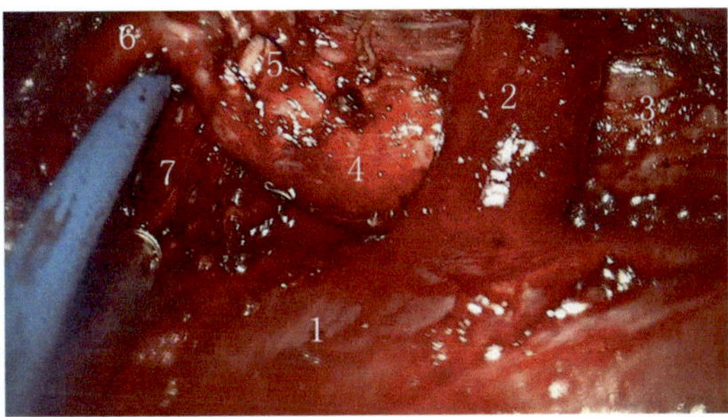

Fig. 2.47 1—Superior vena cava, 2—arch of azygos vein, 3—trachea, 4—right principal bronchus, 5—right superior lobar bronchial stump, 6—right middle segment bronchus, 7—left principal bronchus. After the infracarinal lymph node dissection

Excision of the Middle Lobe of Right Lung

3

The bronchus of the middle lobe of the right lung is located in the depth of the artery, and there are relatively many lymph nodes distributed along the middle lobe bronchus and often fused together. Therefore, lymph node dissection is the key and difficult point in radical resection of the middle lobe lung cancer (Figs. 3.1, 3.2, 3.3, 3.4, 3.5, 3.6, 3.7, 3.8, 3.9, 3.10, 3.11, 3.12, 3.13, 3.14, 3.15, 3.16, 3.17, 3.18, 3.19, 3.20, 3.21, 3.22, 3.23, 3.24, 3.25, 3.26, 3.27, 3.28, 3.29, 3.30, 3.31, 3.32, 3.33, 3.34, 3.35, 3.36, 3.37, and 3.38).

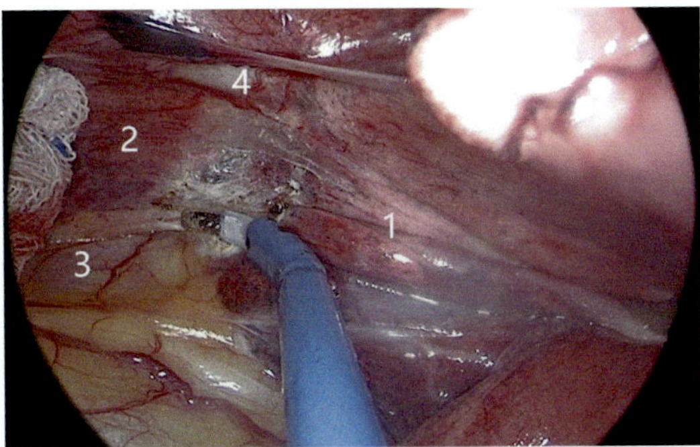

Fig. 3.2 1—Middle lobe of right lung, 2—inferior lobe of right lung, 3—right inferior pulmonary vein, 4—right inferior pulmonary artery. Opening the interlobar fissure

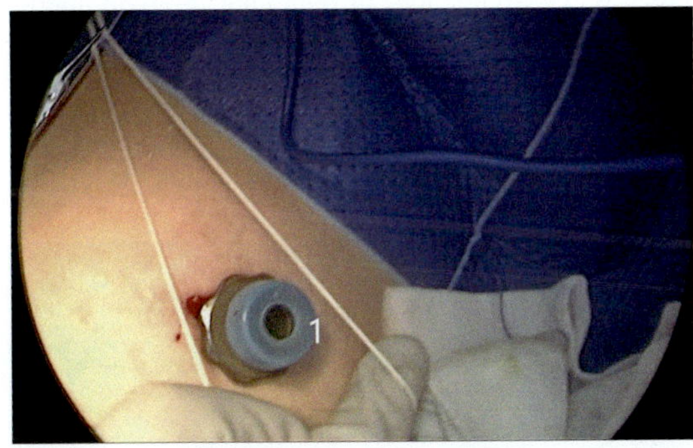

Fig. 3.1 1—Incision trocar. Showing the incision

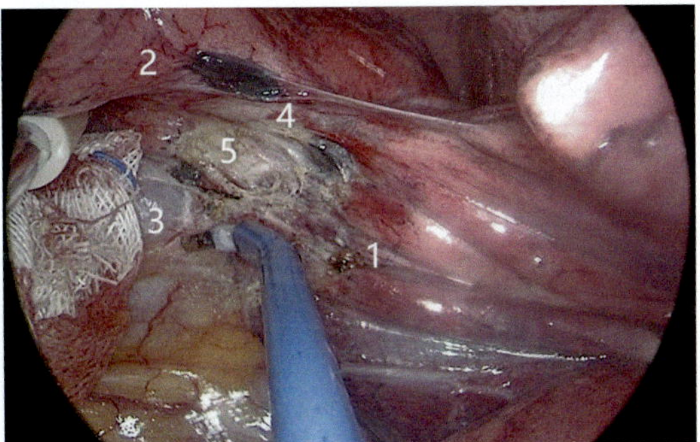

Fig. 3.3 1—Middle lobe of right lung, 2—inferior lobe of right lung, 3—right inferior pulmonary vein, 4—right inferior pulmonary artery, 5—right inferior lobar bronchus. Dissect along the upper right inferior pulmonary vein and reveal the right inferior lobar bronchus

J. Li, Z. Long, *Atlas of Thoracoscopic Lobectomy with Bronchoplasty*,
https://doi.org/10.1007/978-981-99-5150-5_3

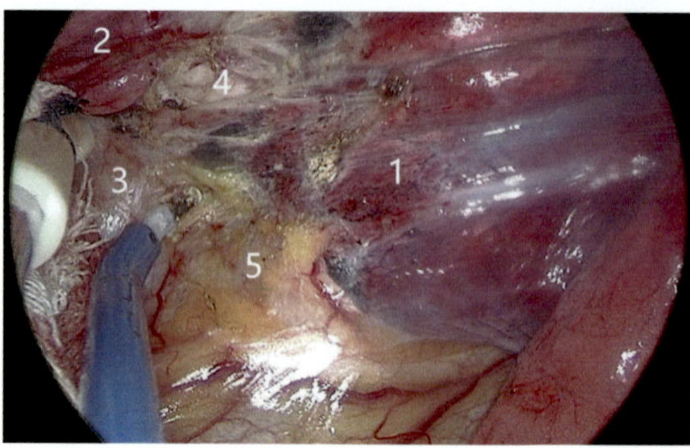

Fig. 3.4 1—Middle lobe of right lung, 2—inferior lobe of right lung, 3—right inferior pulmonary vein, 4—right inferior lobar bronchus, 5—right middle pulmonary vein. Dissect the lymph node above the right inferior pulmonary vein and reveal the right middle pulmonary vein

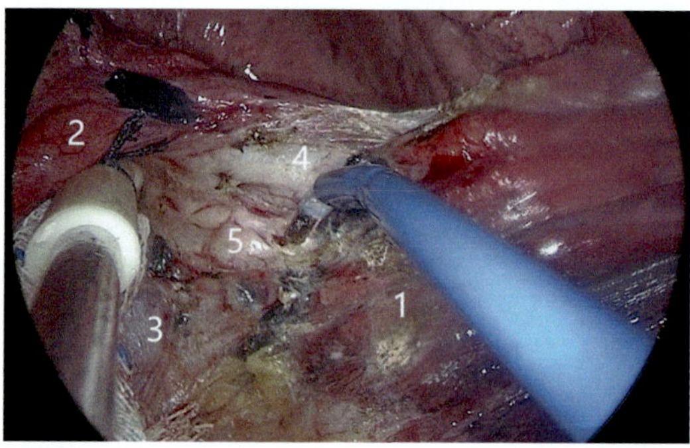

Fig. 3.5 1—Middle lobe of right lung, 2—inferior lobe of right lung, 3—right inferior pulmonary vein, 4—right inferior pulmonary artery, 5—right inferior lobar bronchus. Dissect along the right inferior lobar bronchus upward and dissect the lymph node in front of the right inferior lobar bronchus

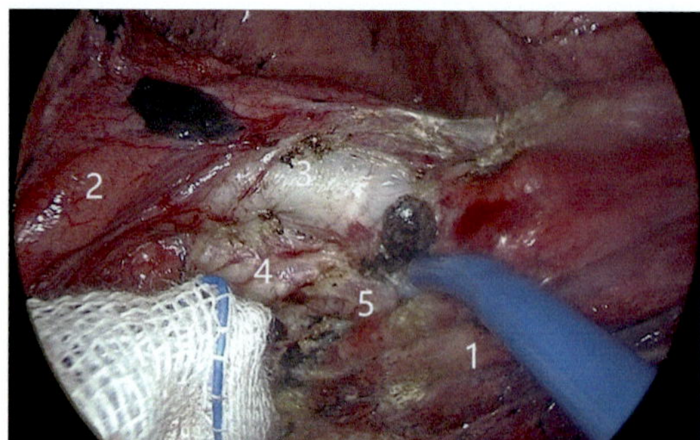

Fig. 3.6 1—Middle lobe of right lung, 2—inferior lobe of right lung, 3—right inferior pulmonary artery, 4—right inferior lobar bronchus, 5—right middle lobar bronchus. Continue to dissect along the right inferior lobar bronchus upward and dissect the lymph node to reveal the right middle lobar bronchus

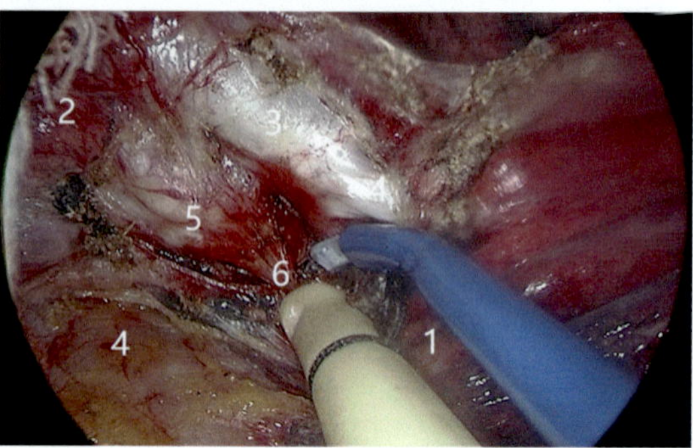

Fig. 3.7 1—Middle lobe of right lung, 2—inferior lobe of right lung, 3—right inferior pulmonary artery, 4—right inferior pulmonary vein, 5—right inferior lobar bronchus, 6—right middle lobar bronchus. Cut the right middle lobar bronchus at the beginning

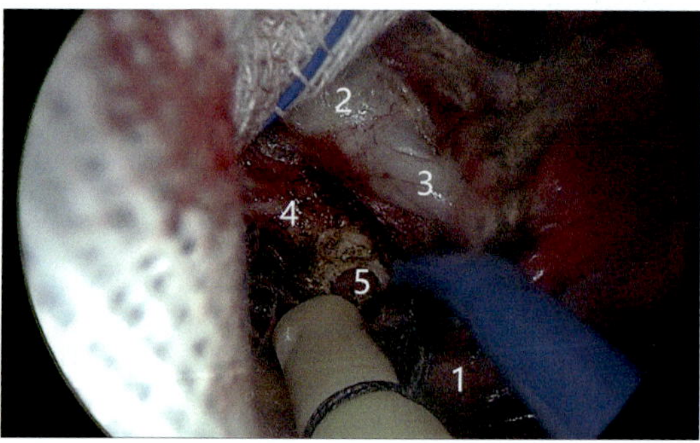

Fig. 3.8 1—Middle lobe of right lung, 2—right inferior pulmonary artery, 3—right middle lobe lateral segment artery, 4—right inferior lobar bronchus, 5—right middle lobar bronchus. Cut the right middle lobar bronchus at the beginning

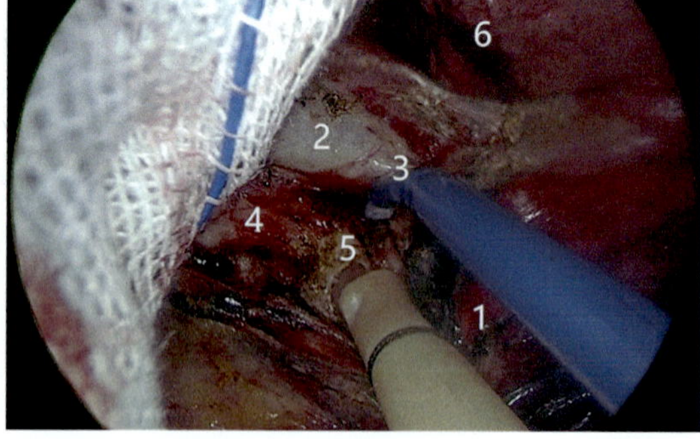

Fig. 3.9 1—Middle lobe of right lung, 2—right inferior pulmonary artery, 3—right middle lobe lateral segment artery, 4—right inferior lobar bronchus, 5—right middle lobar bronchial stump, 6—superior lobe of right lung. Dissect the lymph node between right middle lobe lateral segment artery and bronchus

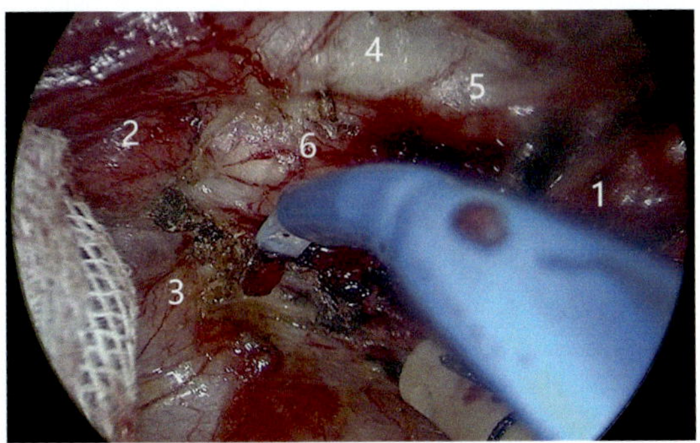

Fig. 3.10 1—Middle lobe of right lung, 2—inferior lobe of right lung, 3—right inferior pulmonary vein, 4—right inferior pulmonary artery, 5—right middle lobe lateral segment artery, 6—right inferior lobar bronchus. Dissect the lymph node beside the right inferior lobar bronchus along the right inferior pulmonary vein upward and backward

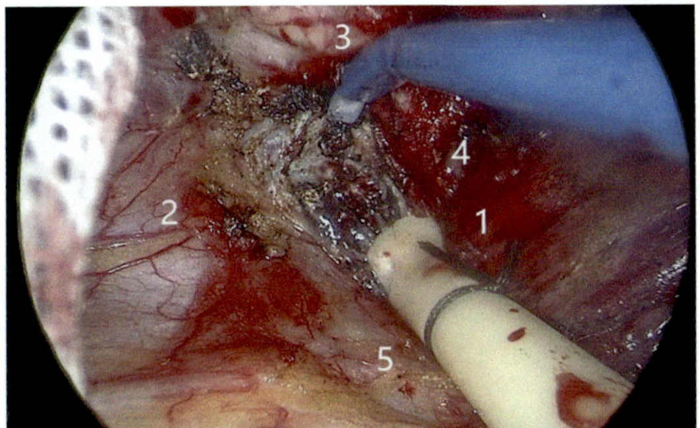

Fig. 3.11 1—Middle lobe of right lung, 2—right inferior pulmonary vein, 3—right inferior lobar bronchus, 4—right middle lobar bronchial stump, 5—right middle pulmonary vein. Continue to dissect the lymph node beside the right inferior lobar bronchus along the right inferior pulmonary vein upward and backward, and connect to the infracarinal lymph node

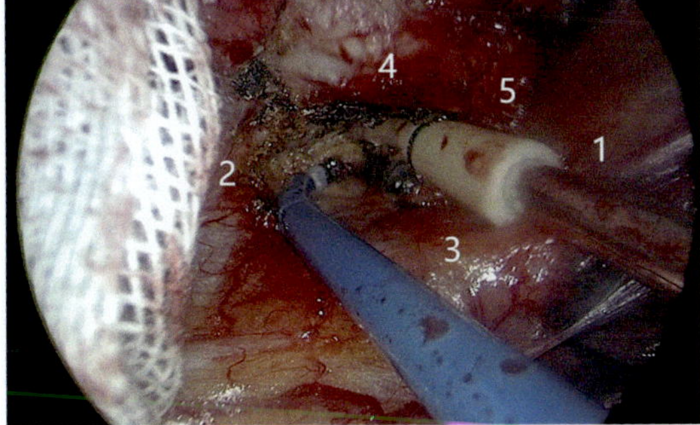

Fig. 3.12 1—Middle lobe of right lung, 2—right inferior pulmonary vein, 3—right middle pulmonary vein, 4—right inferior lobar bronchus, 5—right middle lobar bronchial stump. Dissect the lymph node along the right middle pulmonary vein and posterior pericardium upward and backward

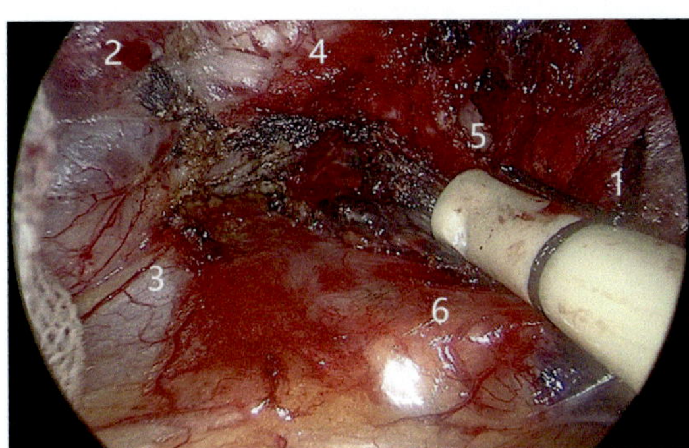

Fig. 3.13 1—Middle lobe of right lung, 2—inferior lobe of right lung, 3—right inferior pulmonary vein, 4—right inferior lobar bronchus, 5—right middle lobar bronchial stump, 6—right middle pulmonary vein. Continue to dissect the lymph node along the right middle pulmonary vein and posterior pericardium upward and backward

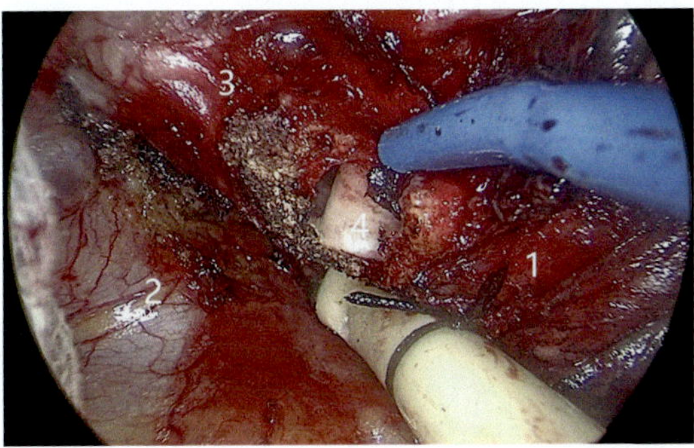

Fig. 3.14 1—Middle lobe of right lung, 2—right inferior pulmonary vein, 3—right inferior lobar bronchus, 4—right middle lobar bronchus opening. Cut off the right middle lobar bronchus along the right middle lobar bronchus opening

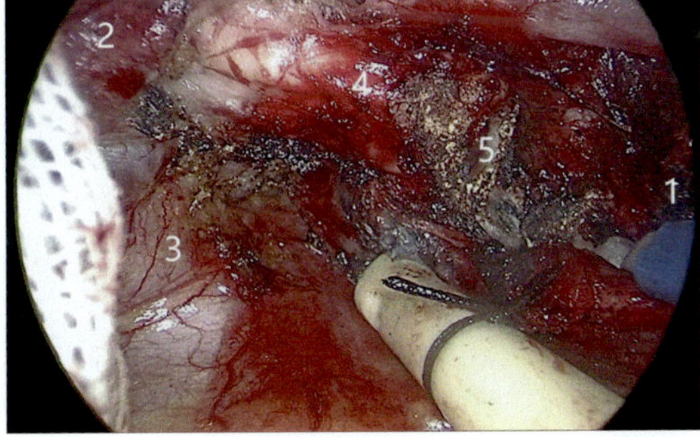

Fig. 3.15 1—Middle lobe of right lung, 2—inferior lobe of right lung, 3—right inferior pulmonary vein, 4—right inferior lobar bronchus, 5—right middle lobar bronchial stump. Dissect the lymph node between the upper right middle lobar bronchus opening and right middle segment bronchus

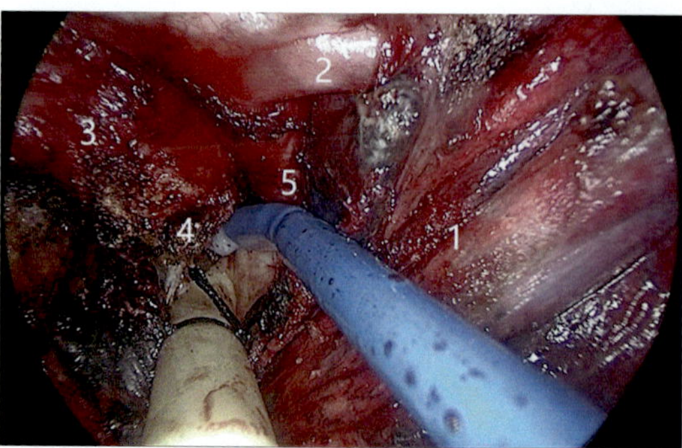

Fig. 3.16 1—Middle lobe of right lung, 2—right middle lobe lateral segment artery, 3—right inferior lobar bronchus, 4—right middle lobar bronchial stump, 5—interlobar trunk of right pulmonary artery. Dissect the lymph node around the right middle lobar bronchus opening downward and backward, and connect to the lymph node dissected before

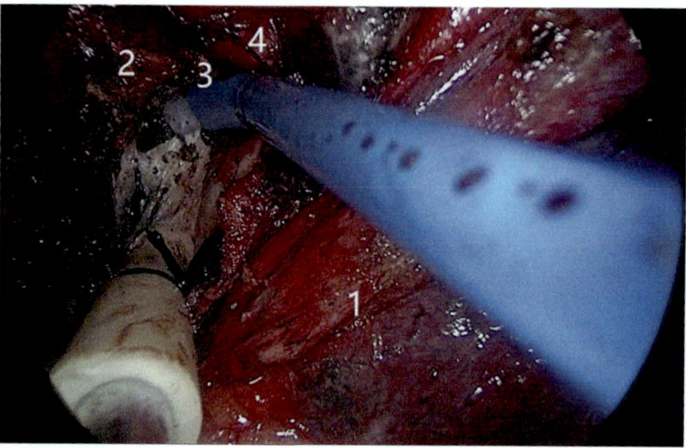

Fig. 3.17 1—Middle lobe of right lung, 2—right inferior lobar bronchus, 3—right middle lobar bronchial stump, 4—right middle lobe lateral segment artery. Dissect the lymph node which is inner rear the right middle lobar bronchus along the right middle lobar bronchus opening upward and backward

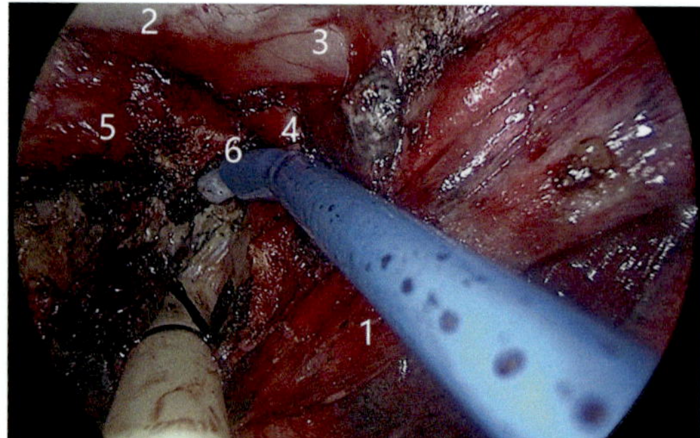

Fig. 3.18 1—Middle lobe of right lung, 2—right inferior pulmonary artery, 3—right middle lobe lateral segment artery, 4—interlobar trunk of right pulmonary artery, 5—right inferior lobar bronchus, 6—right middle lobar bronchial stump. Dissect the lymph node behind the right middle lobar bronchus

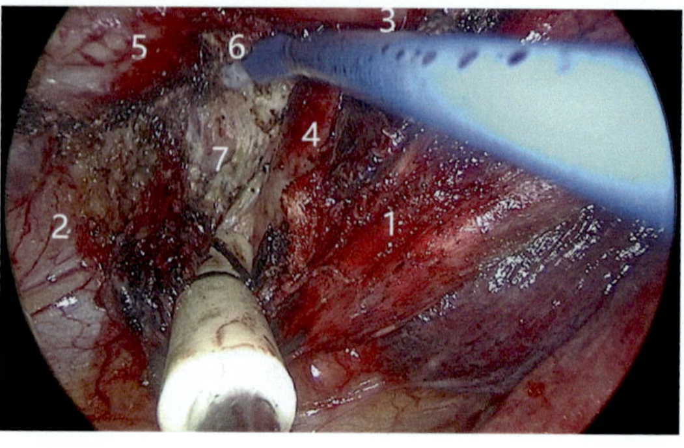

Fig. 3.19 1—Middle lobe of right lung, 2—right inferior pulmonary vein, 3—right middle lobe lateral segment artery, 4—interlobar trunk of right pulmonary artery, 5—right inferior lobar bronchus, 6—right middle lobar bronchial stump, 7—esophagus. Dissect the lymph node behind the right middle lobar bronchus to anterior esophagus and reveal esophagus

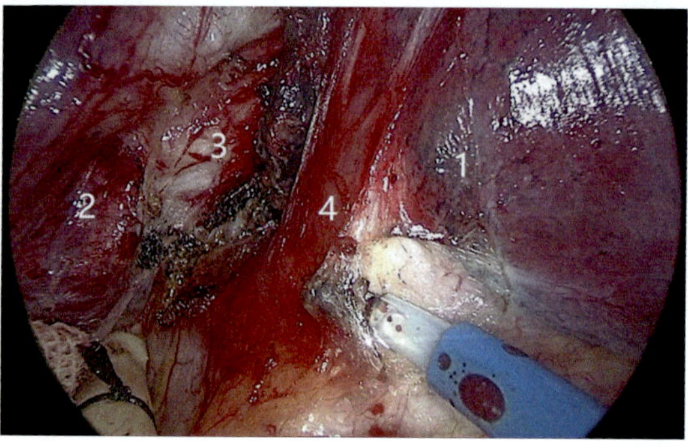

Fig. 3.20 1—Superior lobe of right lung, 2—inferior lobe of right lung, 3—right inferior lobar bronchus, 4—right middle pulmonary vein. Dissect from the anterior right inferior pulmonary vein downward and reveal the right middle pulmonary vein

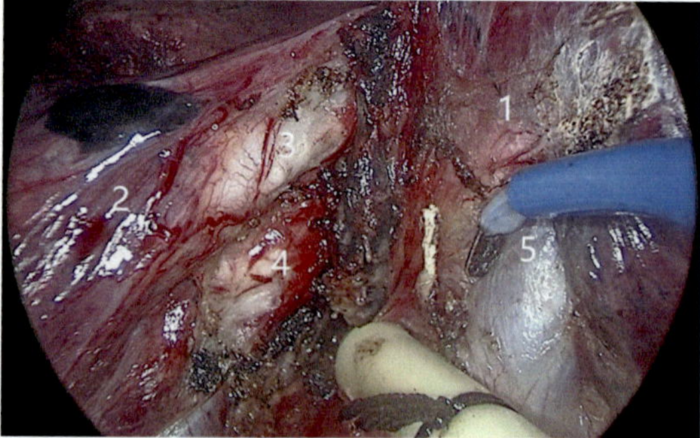

Fig. 3.21 1—Superior lobe of right lung, 2—inferior lobe of right lung, 3—right inferior pulmonary artery, 4—right inferior lobar bronchus, 5—right middle pulmonary vein. Dissect the lymph node behind the right middle pulmonary vein

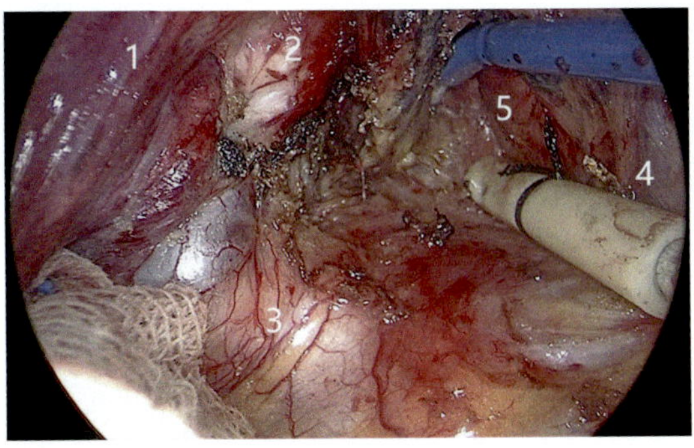

Fig. 3.22 1—Inferior lobe of right lung, 2—right inferior lobar bronchus, 3—right inferior pulmonary vein, 4—right middle pulmonary vein, 5—interlobar trunk of right pulmonary artery. Continue to dissect the lymph node along the right middle pulmonary vein backward, and dissect the lymph node of interlobar trunk of right pulmonary artery and posterior pericardium

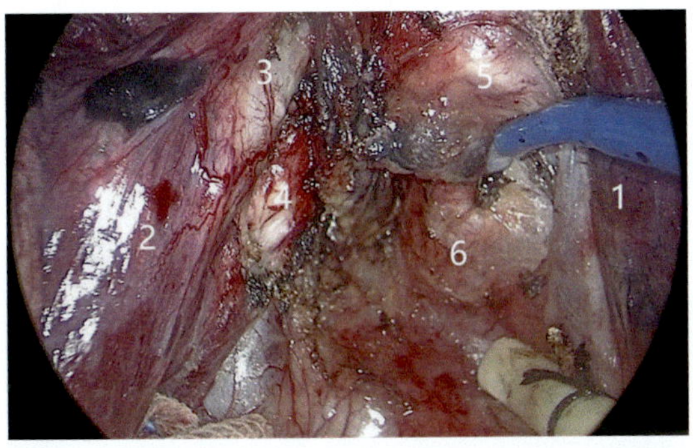

Fig. 3.23 1—Superior lobe of right lung, 2—inferior lobe of right lung, 3—right inferior pulmonary artery, 4—right inferior lobar bronchus, 5—right middle lobar bronchus, 6—interlobar trunk of right pulmonary artery. Dissect the lymph node along the anterior interlobar trunk of right pulmonary artery far away

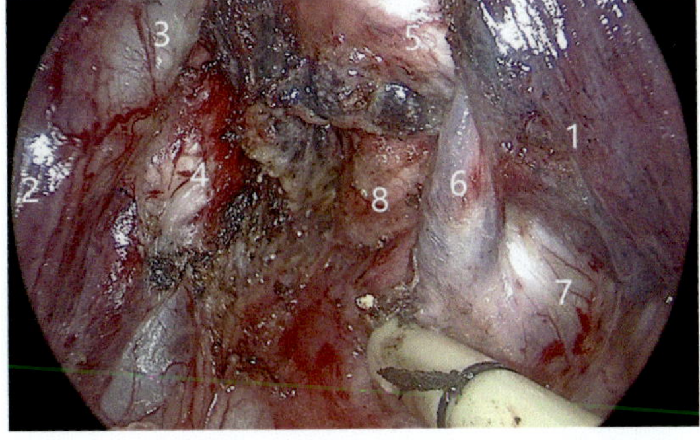

Fig. 3.24 1—Superior lobe of right lung, 2—inferior lobe of right lung, 3—right inferior pulmonary artery, 4—right inferior lobar bronchus, 5—right middle lobar bronchus, 6—right middle pulmonary vein, 7—right superior pulmonary vein, 8—interlobar trunk of right pulmonary artery. Dissection is finished

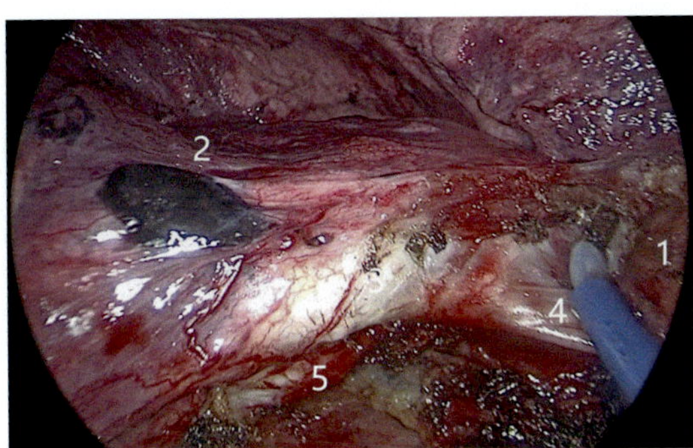

Fig. 3.25 1—Superior lobe of right lung, 2—inferior lobe of right lung, 3—right inferior pulmonary artery, 4—right middle lobe lateral segment artery, 5—right inferior lobar bronchus. Dissect the posterior right middle lobe lateral segment artery

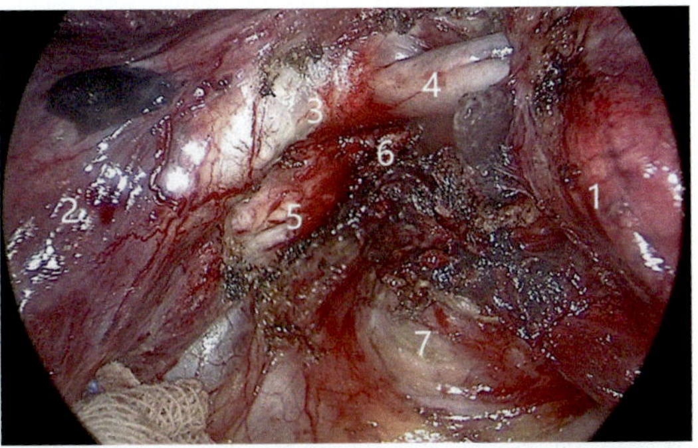

Fig. 3.26 1—Superior lobe of right lung, 2—inferior lobe of right lung, 3—right inferior pulmonary artery, 4—right middle lobe lateral segment artery, 5—right inferior lobar bronchus, 5—right middle lobar bronchus, 6—right middle lobar bronchial stump, 7—right superior pulmonary vein. Dissect the right middle lobe lateral segment artery completely

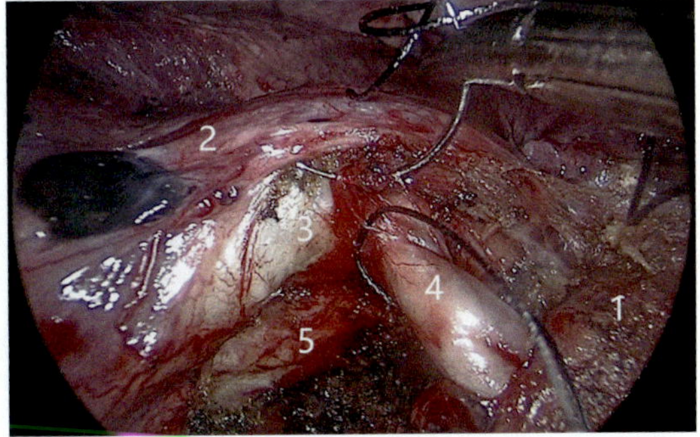

Fig. 3.27 1—Middle lobe of right lung, 2—inferior lobe of right lung, 3—right inferior pulmonary artery, 4—right middle lobe lateral segment artery, 5—right inferior lobar bronchus. Suture and interrupt the right middle lobe lateral segment artery

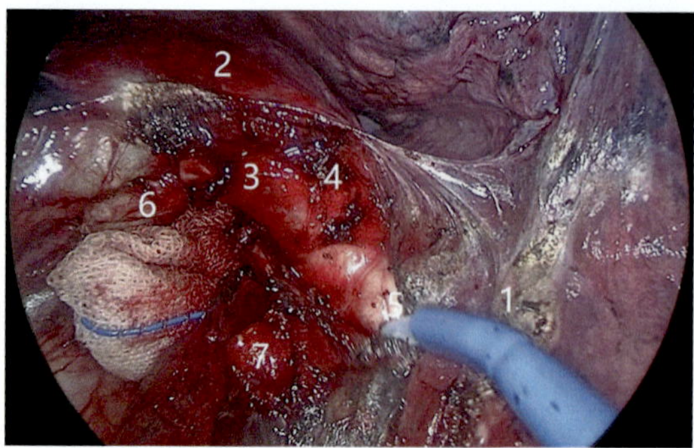

Fig. 3.28 1—Middle lobe of right lung, 2—inferior lobe of right lung, 3—right middle lobe lateral segment artery stump, 4—interlobar trunk of right pulmonary artery, 5—right middle lobe medial segment artery, 6—right inferior lobar bronchus, 7—right middle lobar bronchial stump. Dissected above the right middle lobe lateral segment artery along the interlobar trunk of right pulmonary artery upward and inward to reveal the right middle lobe medial segment artery

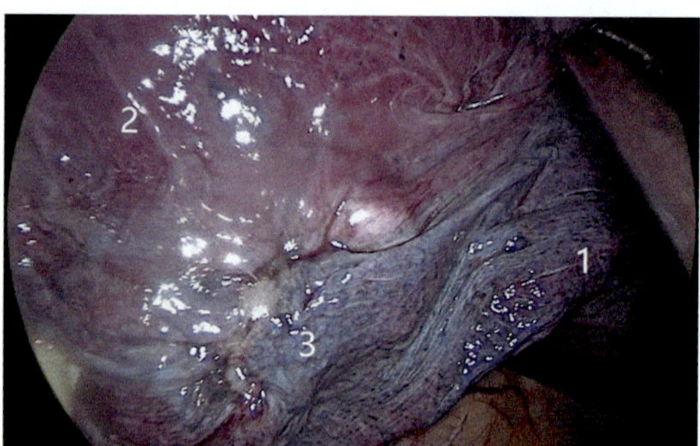

Fig. 3.29 1—Superior lobe of right lung, 2—middle lobe of right lung, 3—tumor in the middle lobe of right lung. Reveal the tumor in the middle lobe of the right lung

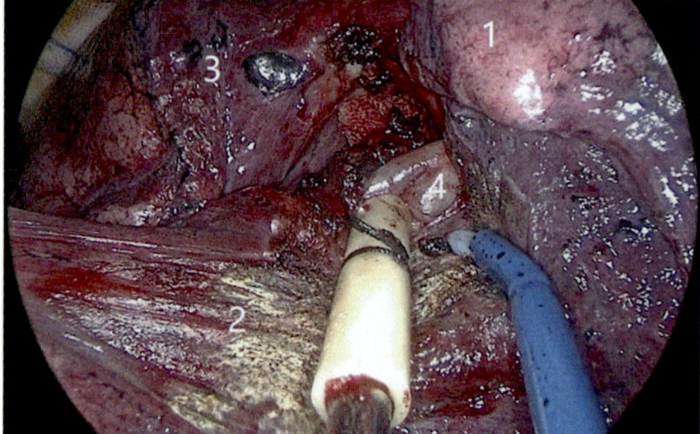

Fig. 3.30 1—Superior lobe of right lung, 2—middle lobe of right lung, 3—inferior lobe of right lung, 4—right middle lobe medial segment artery. Opening the interlobar fissure with an electrotome to reveal the medial segment of the right middle lobe artery

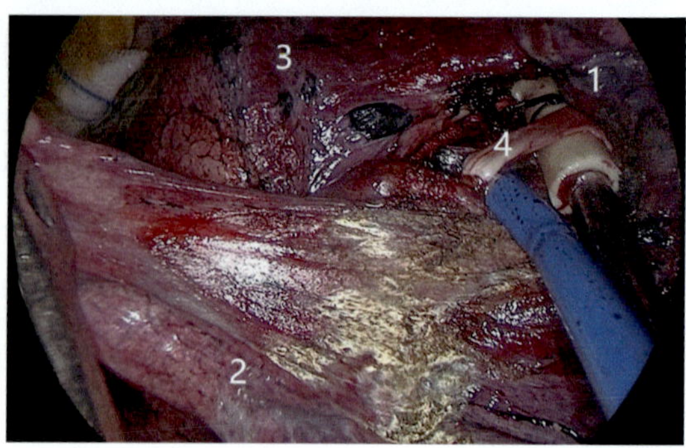

Fig. 3.31 1—Superior lobe of right lung, 2—middle lobe of right lung, 3—inferior lobe of right lung, 4—right middle lobe medial segment artery branch. Cut off the right middle lobe medial segment artery branch with an electrotome

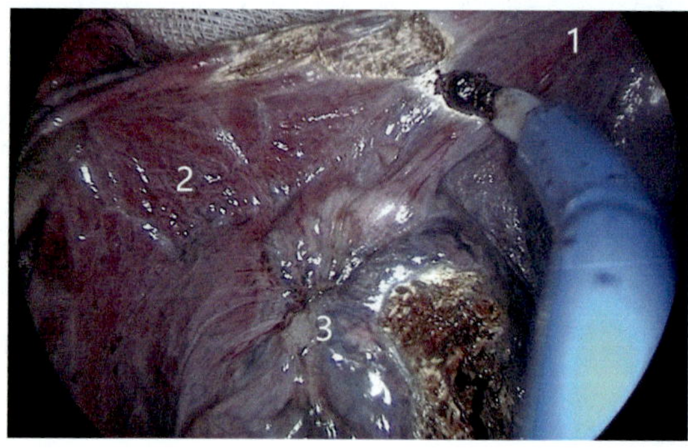

Fig. 3.32 1—Superior lobe of right lung, 2—middle lobe of right lung, 3—tumor in the middle lobe of right lung. Far from tumor in the middle lobe of right lung, resect partial superior lobe of right lung

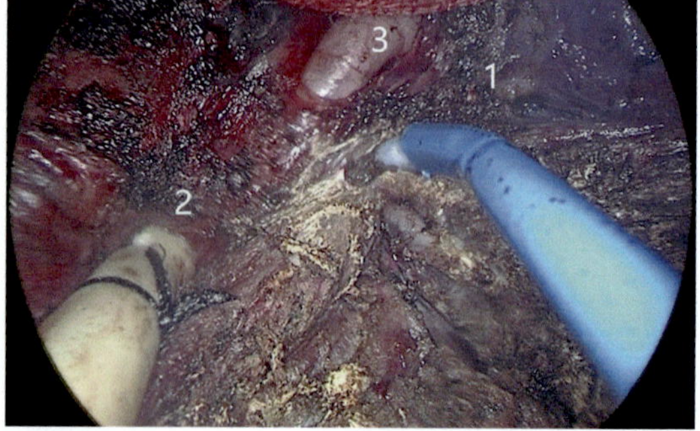

Fig. 3.33 1—Superior lobe of right lung, 2—middle lobe of right lung, 3—right middle lobe medial segment artery branch. Excise interlobar fissure, reveal medial segment of the right middle lobe artery

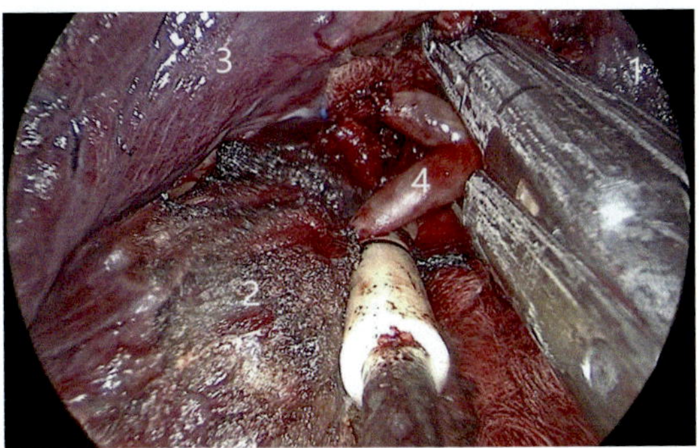

Fig. 3.34 1—Superior lobe of right lung, 2—middle lobe of right lung, 3—inferior lobe of right lung, 4—right middle lobe medial segment artery branch. Cut off the medial segment of the right middle lobe artery with GIA

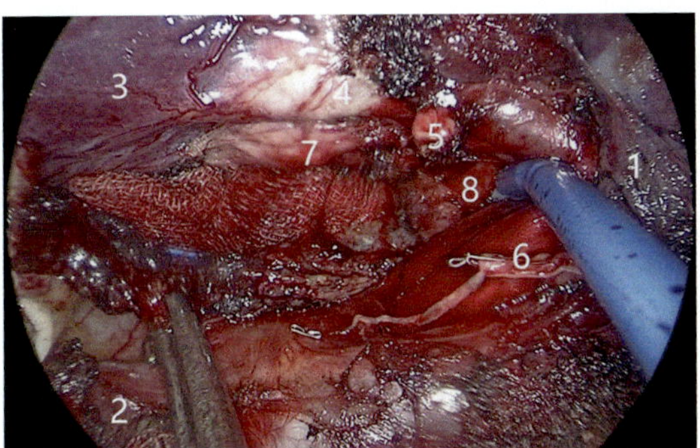

Fig. 3.35 1—Superior lobe of right lung, 2—middle lobe of right lung, 3—inferior lobe of right lung, 4—right inferior pulmonary artery, 5—lateral segment stump of right inferior pulmonary artery, 6—right middle lobe medial segment artery stump, 7—right inferior lobar bronchus, 8—left principal bronchus. Dissect the infracarinal lymph node along the posterior interlobar trunk of right pulmonary artery

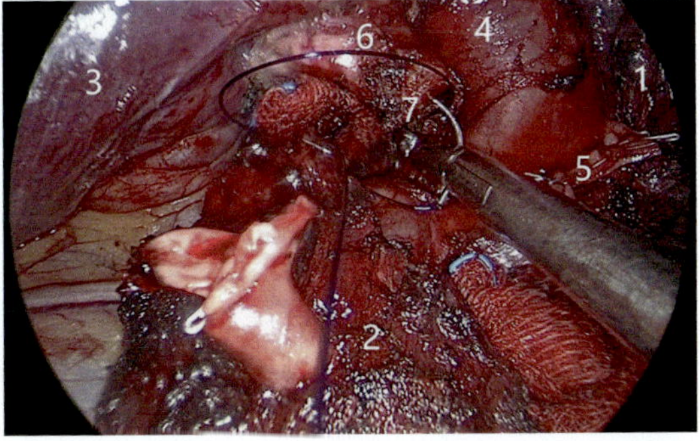

Fig. 3.36 1—Superior lobe of right lung, 2—middle lobe of right lung, 3—inferior lobe of right lung, 4—right inferior pulmonary artery, 5—right middle lobe medial segment artery stump, 6—right inferior lobar bronchus, 7—right middle lobar bronchial stump. Take continuous suture of right middle lobar bronchial stump

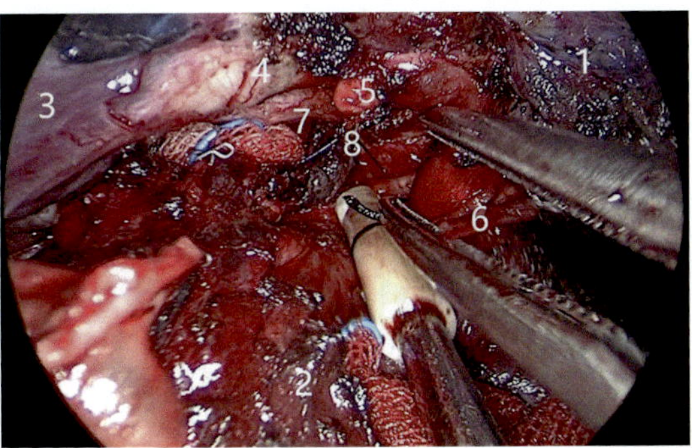

Fig. 3.37 1—Superior lobe of right lung, 2—middle lobe of right lung, 3—inferior lobe of right lung, 4—right inferior pulmonary artery, 5—lateral segment stump of right inferior pulmonary artery, 6—right middle lobe medial segment artery stump, 7—right inferior lobar bronchus, 8—right middle lobar bronchial stump. Dissect the infracarinal lymph node along left principal bronchus downward

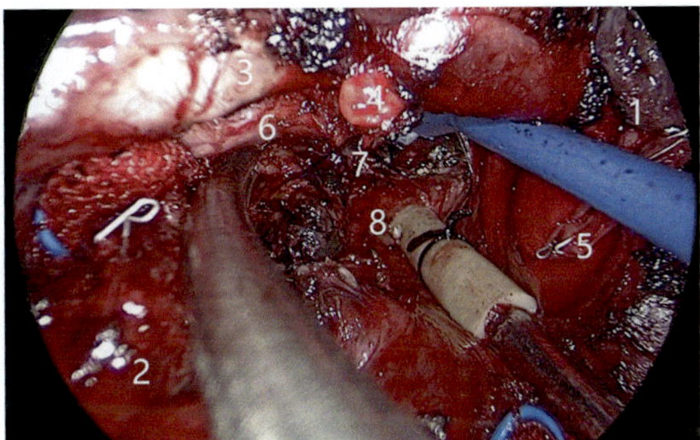

Fig. 3.38 1—Superior lobe of right lung, 2—middle lobe of right lung, 3—right inferior pulmonary artery, 4—lateral segment stump of right inferior pulmonary artery, 5—right middle lobe medial segment artery stump, 6—right inferior lobar bronchus, 7—right middle lobar bronchial stump, 8—left principal bronchus. Dissect the lymph node along right principal bronchus and right middle lobar bronchus, and infracarinal lymph node dissection is finished

Lymph node dissection starts from above the lower lobe vein of the left lung, and sweeps up along the lower lobe bronchus to expose the opening of the middle bronchus. The middle bronchus is cut open at the opening, so that the tissues around the middle bronchus are more easily dissociated, which is conducive to complete removal of the lymph nodes around the bronchus. It is necessary to have a spatial concept to cut off the middle bronchus, the lower bronchus and the middle bronchus form different angles. During the operation, attention should be paid to the Angle changes to cut off horizontally. After cutting off the middle bronchus, the middle trachea and the carina can be exposed behind and above, and the lymph nodes under the carina can be cleaned from the front (Figs. 3.39, 3.40, 3.41, 3.42, 3.43, 3.44, 3.45, 3.46, 3.47, 3.48, 3.49, 3.50, 3.51, 3.52, 3.53, 3.54, and 3.55).

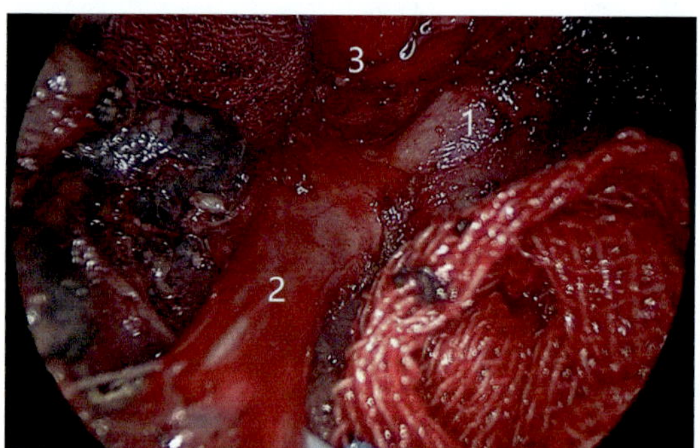

Fig. 3.39 1—Right superior pulmonary vein, 2—right middle pulmonary vein, 3—interlobar trunk of right pulmonary artery. Reveal the right middle pulmonary vein

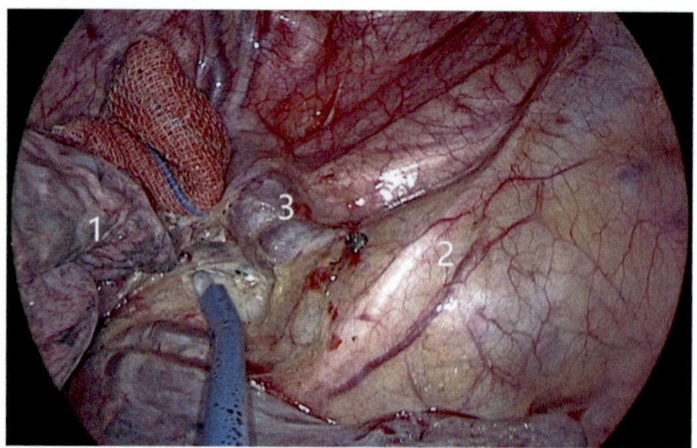

Fig. 3.40 1—Superior lobe of right lung, 2—superior vena cava, 3—arch of azygos vein. Open the adventitia of anterior trunk of right superior lobar artery

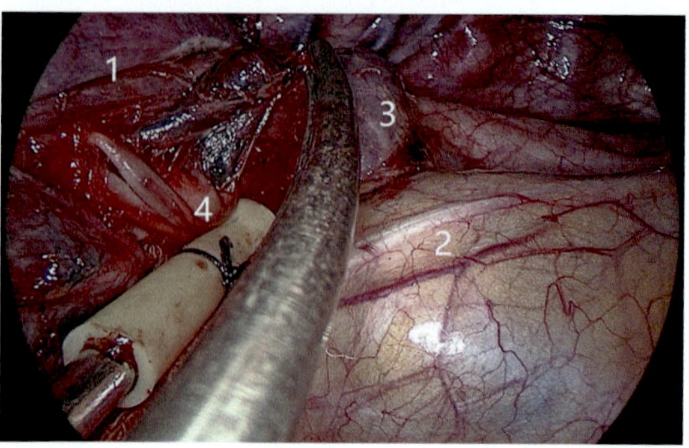

Fig. 3.41 1—Superior lobe of right lung, 2—superior vena cava, 3—arch of azygos vein, 4—anterior trunk of right superior lobar artery. Dissect the hilar lymph node

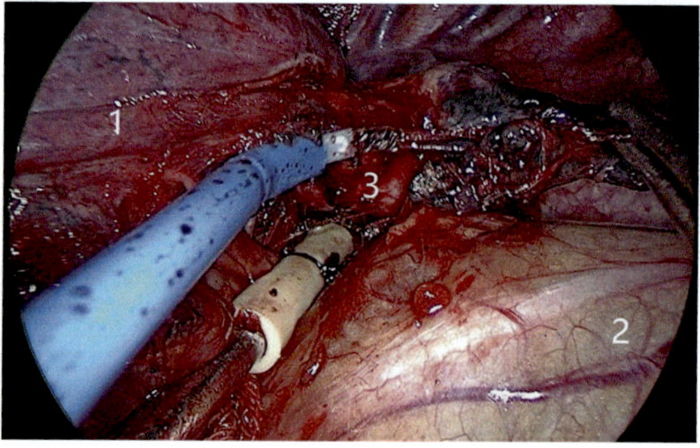

Fig. 3.42 1—Superior lobe of right lung, 2—superior vena cava, 3—beginning of right superior lobar bronchus. The lymph and connective tissues between the inferior arch of azygos vein and superior anterior trunk of right superior lobar artery are completely resected

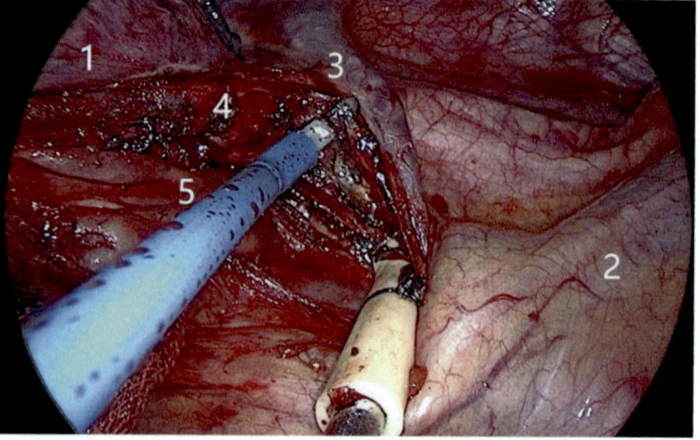

Fig. 3.43 1—Superior lobe of right lung, 2—superior vena cava, 3—arch of azygos vein, 4—right superior lobar bronchus, 5—anterior trunk of right superior lobar artery. Dissect the lymph node along the posterior arch of azygos vein

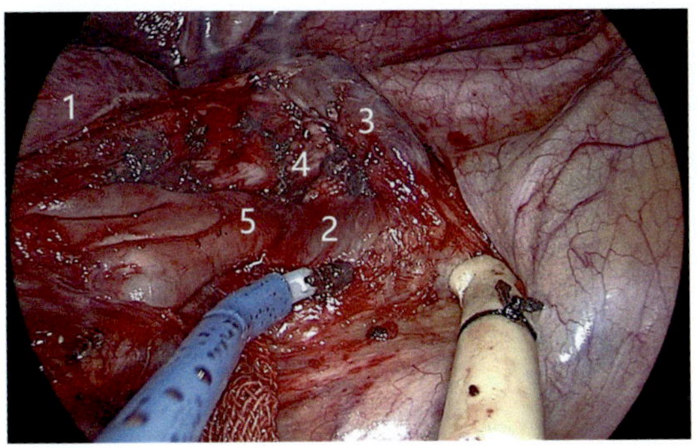

Fig. 3.44 1—Superior lobe of right lung, 2—superior vena cava, 3—arch of azygos vein, 4—right principal bronchus, 5—anterior trunk of right superior lobar artery. Dissect the lymph node along the posterior superior vena cava

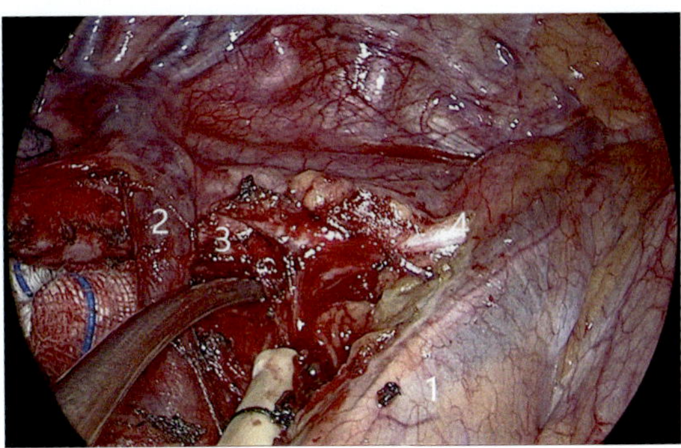

Fig. 3.47 1—Superior vena cava, 2—arch of azygos vein, 3—trachea, 4—right vagus. Dissect the lymph node along the anterior trachea and inferior vagus

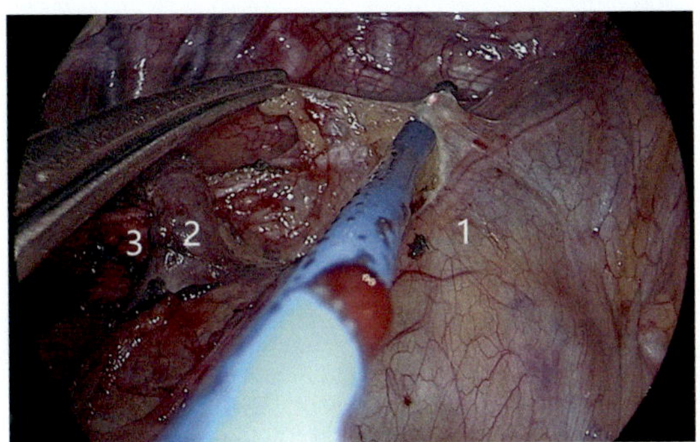

Fig. 3.45 1—Superior vena cava, 2—arch of azygos vein, 3—right principal bronchus. Open the mediastinum pleura behind the superior vena cava

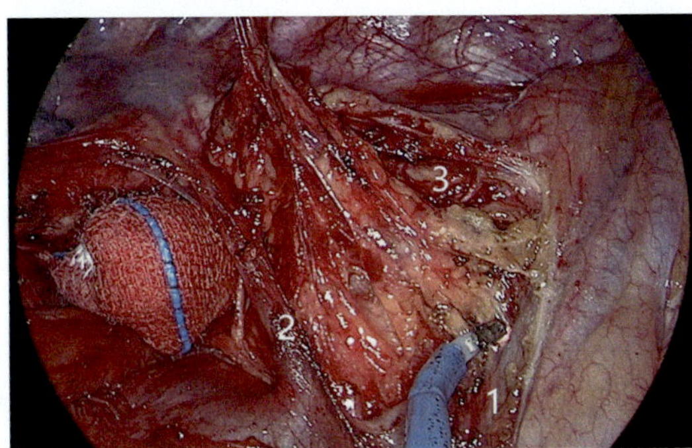

Fig. 3.48 1—Superior vena cava, 2—arch of azygos vein, 3—right vagus. Dissect the lymph node along posterior superior vena cava upward to inferior right innominate vein

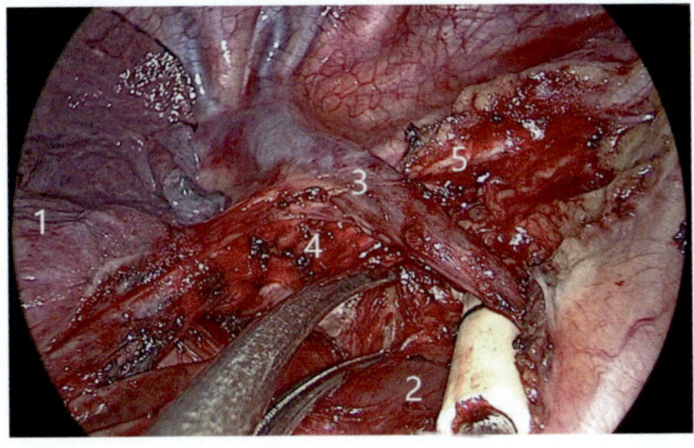

Fig. 3.46 1—Superior lobe of right lung, 2—superior vena cava, 3—arch of azygos vein, 4—right principal bronchus, 5—right vagus. Dissect the lymph node along the surface of pericardium

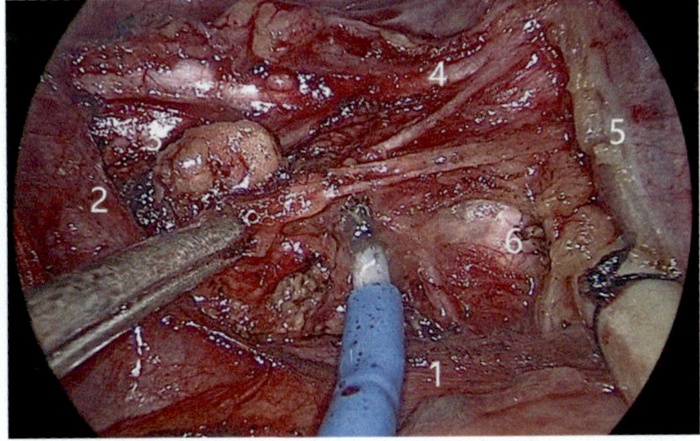

Fig. 3.49 1—Superior vena cava, 2—arch of azygos vein, 3—trachea, 4—right vagus, 5—right innominate vein, 6—right subclavian artery. Dissect the lymph node along right innominate vein downward to reveal right subclavian artery

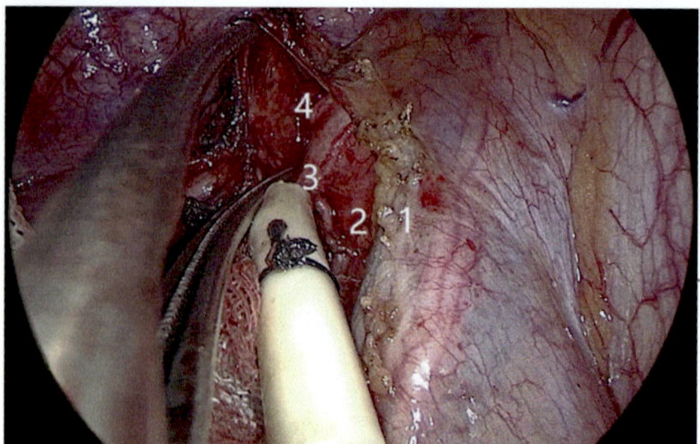

Fig. 3.50 1—Superior vena cava, 2—right subclavian artery, 3—right vagus, 4—right recurrent laryngeal nerve. Reveal right recurrent laryngeal nerve

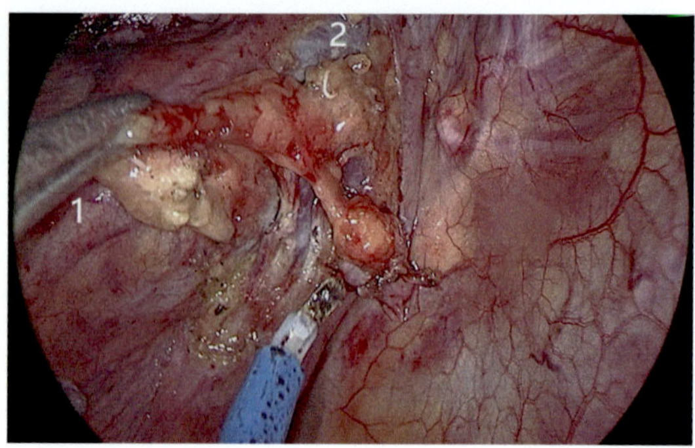

Fig. 3.53 1—Superior vena cava, 2—innominate vein. Dissect 3A lymph node

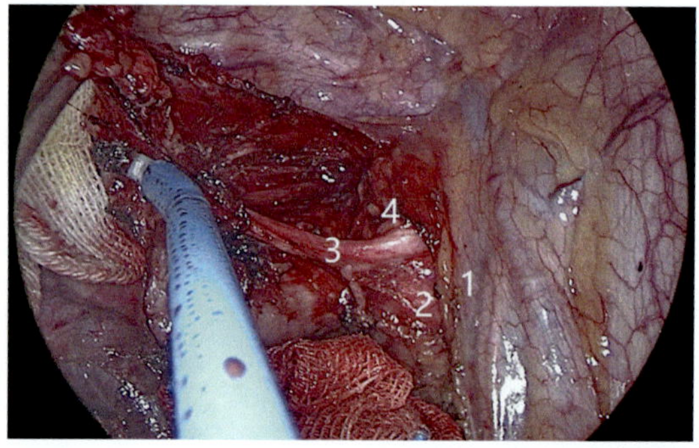

Fig. 3.51 1—Superior vena cava, 2—right subclavian artery, 3—right vagus, 4—right recurrent laryngeal nerve. Dissect the lymph node of vagus and posterior recurrent laryngeal nerve

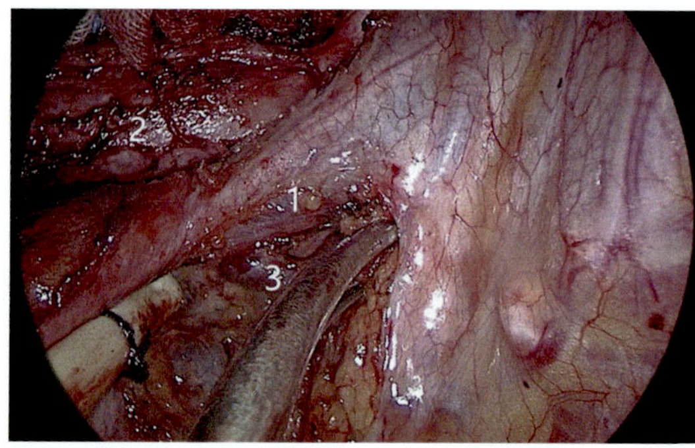

Fig. 3.54 1—Innominate vein, 2—trachea, 3—right internal mammary vein. Dissect 3A lymph node

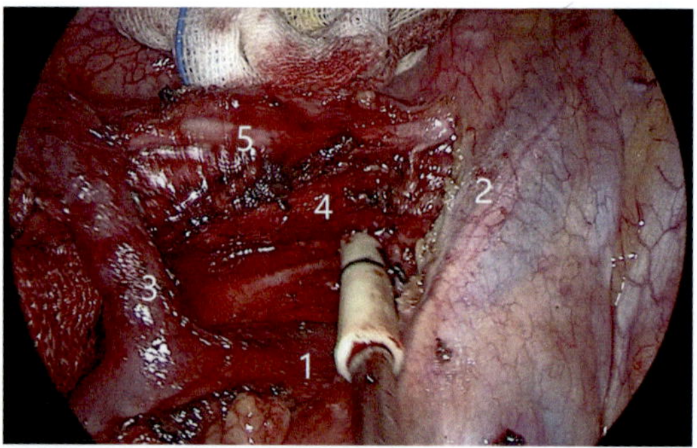

Fig. 3.52 1—Superior vena cava, 2—right innominate vein, 3—arch of azygos vein, 4—trachea, 5—right vagus. Dissection is finished

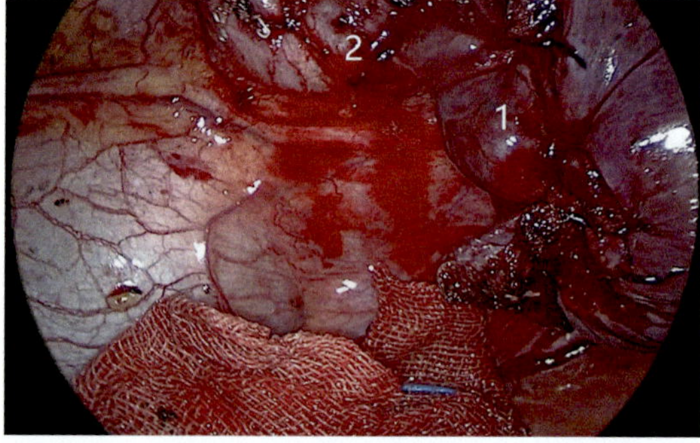

Fig. 3.55 1—Superior lobe of right lung, 2—right superior pulmonary vein. Suture superior lobe stump of right lung

Suture superior lobe stump of right lung. Interrupt the right middle pulmonary vein and remove the specimen.

Summary: The lymph nodes around the middle lobe bronchi are numerous, and complete dissection of the lymph nodes in the drainage area to which the middle lobe tumor belongs is a key factor in determining the success of the operation. In this case, the dissection was started from the anterior aspect of the lower lobe vein, revealing the basal branch of the right lower lobe pulmonary artery and the right lower lobe bronchi that resides anteriorly, and the lymph nodes behind the pericardium were removed at the same time to complete the dissection below the middle lobe bronchi, and the dissection was done upward along the lower lobe bronchi to reveal the opening of the middle lobe bronchus. The middle lobe bronchus is cut at the beginning of the middle lobe bronchus to reveal the lymph nodes behind and above the trachea, which are removed; the middle lobe vein of the right lung is dissociated to reveal the lymph nodes in front of the middle lobe bronchus, which are removed, thus completing the dissection of the entire circumferential lymph nodes of the middle lobe bronchus.

The key to removing the subcarinal lymph nodes from between the veins of the upper and lower lobes of the right lung is to have a good concept of space, and the surgical technique requires a high degree of skill, which can be appreciated by the reader by referring to the chapter on the dissection of subcarinal lymph nodes in the upper lobe of the right lung. Because of the small space, it is especially important to determine the location of the carinal. First, start from the posterior aspect of the pericardium, reveal the anterior aspect of the esophagus, then remove the lymph nodes behind the pericardium along the posterior aspect of the right interlobular trunk of the right pulmonary artery, remove upward along the middle segment of the bronchus, reveal the left main bronchus, remove the lymph nodes below its anterior aspect, and remove downward along the middle segment of the bronchus to complete the subcarinal lymph node dissection.

4 Superior Lobe of Left Lung

Thoracoscopic resection of the left upper lobe of the lung is often considered to be one of the more difficult lobectomies, with many arterial branches and large variation, and the anterior trunk is often thick and short when separated, which is easy to cause damage and cause massive bleeding. Radical resection of lung cancer in the left upper lobe of the lung was performed from the third intercostal space, demonstrating different methods and ideas (Figs. 4.1, 4.2, 4.3, 4.4, 4.5, 4.6, 4.7, 4.8, 4.9, 4.10, 4.11, 4.12, 4.13, 4.14, 4.15, 4.16, 4.17, 4.18, 4.19, 4.20, 4.21, 4.22, 4.23, 4.24, 4.25, 4.26, and 4.27).

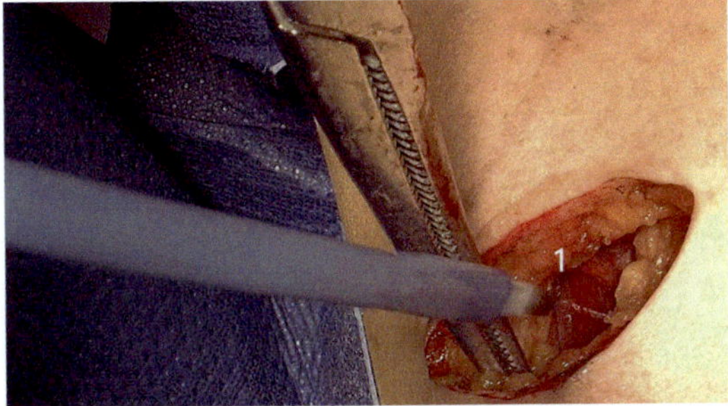

Fig. 4.2 1—Incision. Cut muscle along muscle space

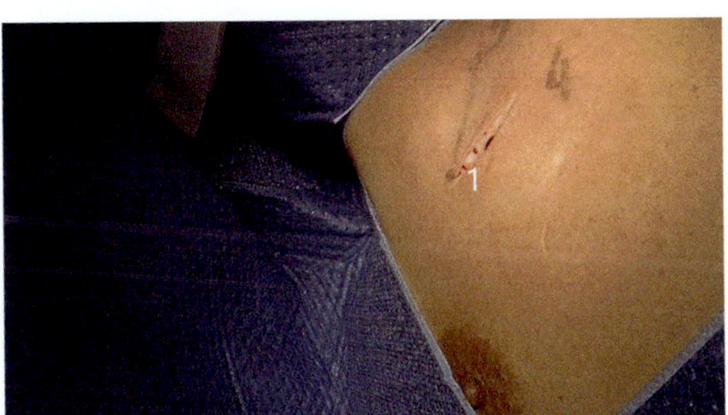

Fig. 4.1 1—Incision. The incision is chosen at anterior axillary line in the third intercostal space

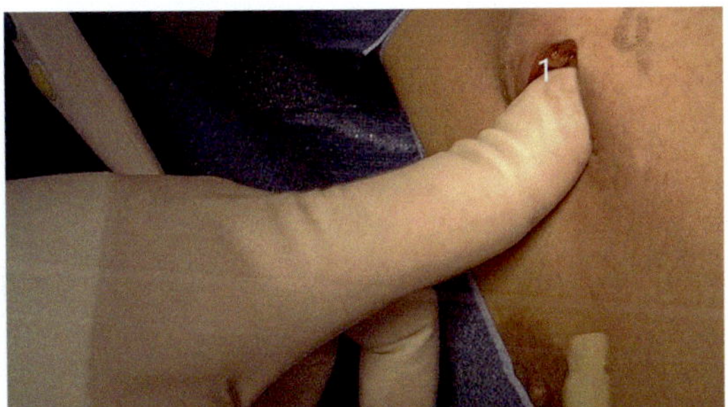

Fig. 4.3 1—Incision. Take blunt dissection of incision with fingers

J. Li, Z. Long, *Atlas of Thoracoscopic Lobectomy with Bronchoplasty*,
https://doi.org/10.1007/978-981-99-5150-5_4

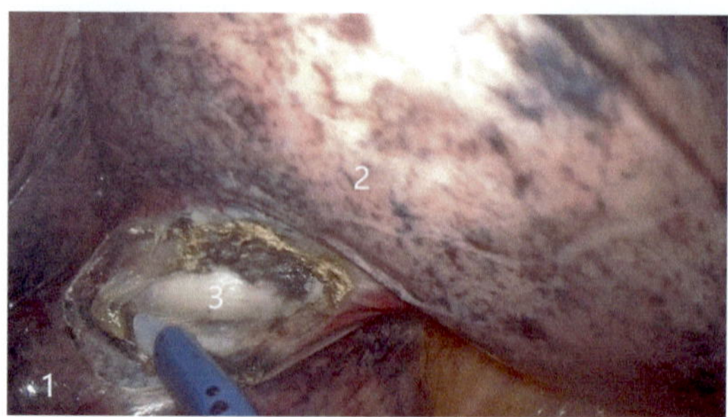

Fig. 4.4 1—Superior lobe of left lung, 2—inferior lobe of left lung, 3—left inferior pulmonary artery. Open the interlobar fissure and reveal left inferior pulmonary artery branch

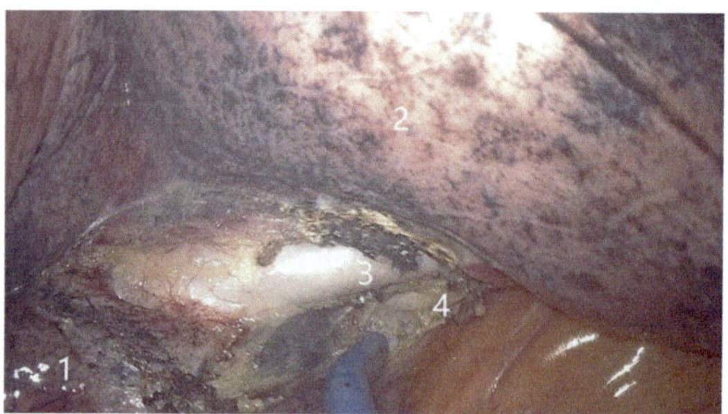

Fig. 4.5 1—Superior lobe of left lung, 2—inferior lobe of left lung, 3—left inferior pulmonary artery, 4—left inferior lobar bronchus. Open the interlobar fissure forward and reveal left inferior lobar bronchus

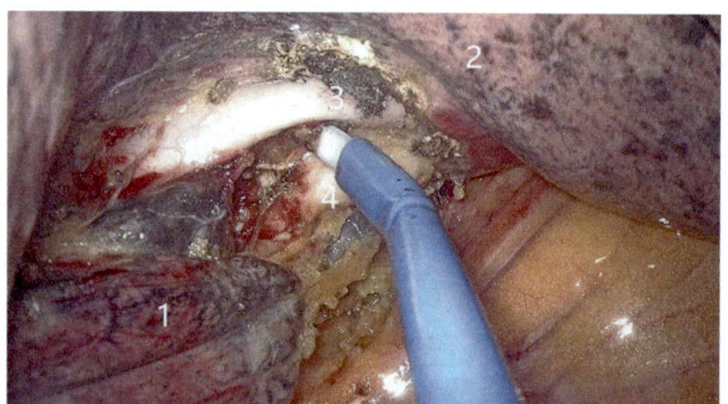

Fig. 4.6 1—Superior lobe of left lung, 2—inferior lobe of left lung, 3—left inferior pulmonary artery, 4—left inferior lobar bronchus. Dissect lymph node between left inferior pulmonary artery and left inferior lobar bronchus

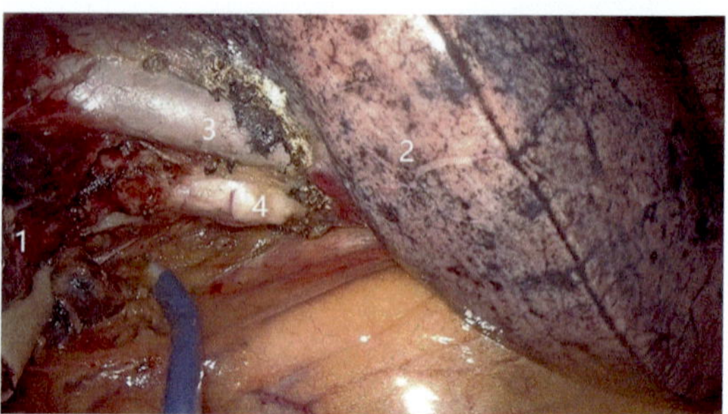

Fig. 4.7 1—Superior lobe of left lung, 2—inferior lobe of left lung, 3—left inferior pulmonary artery, 4—left inferior lobar bronchus. Dissect lymph node behind and below left inferior pulmonary artery

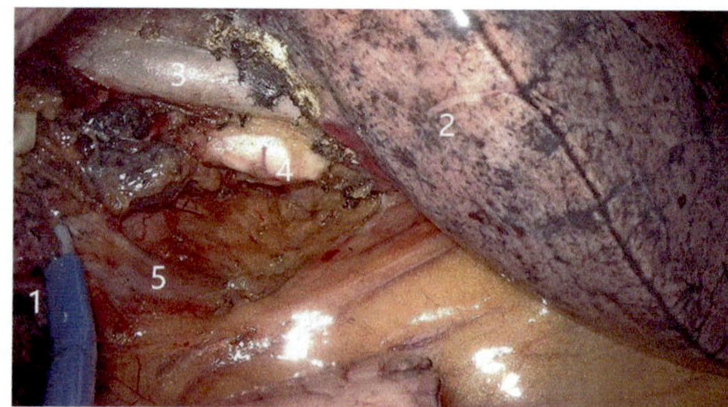

Fig. 4.8 1—Superior lobe of left lung, 2—inferior lobe of left lung, 3—left inferior pulmonary artery, 4—left inferior lobar bronchus, 5—left superior pulmonary vein. Dissect lymph node along anterior left superior pulmonary vein

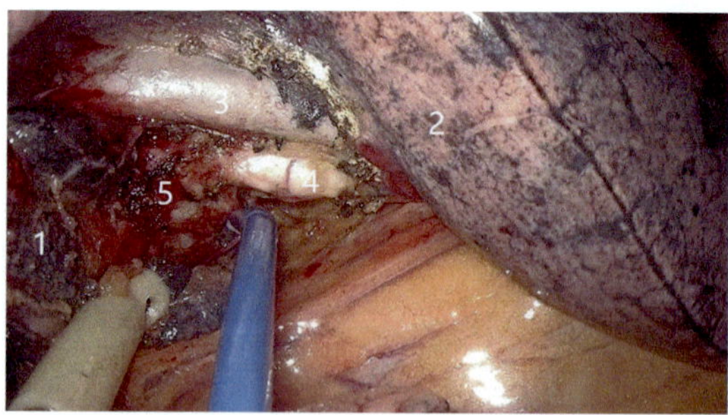

Fig. 4.9 1—Superior lobe of left lung, 2—inferior lobe of left lung, 3—left inferior pulmonary artery, 4—left inferior lobar bronchus, 5—left superior lobar bronchus. Dissect lymph node along left inferior lobar bronchus upward to reveal left superior lobar bronchus

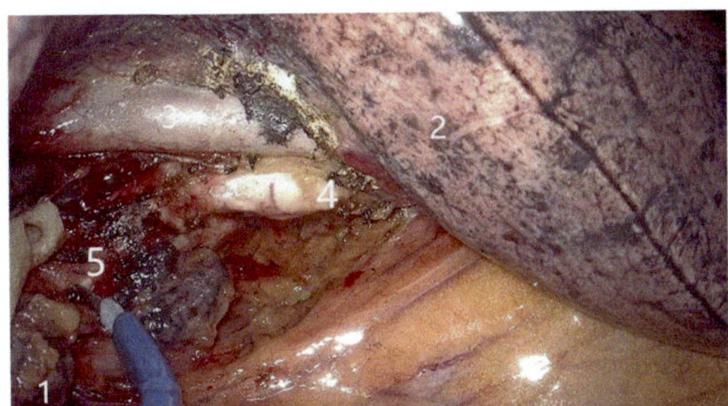

Fig. 4.10 1—Superior lobe of left lung, 2—inferior lobe of left lung, 3—left inferior pulmonary artery, 4—left inferior lobar bronchus, 5—left superior lobar bronchus. Cut at the opening of left superior lobar bronchus

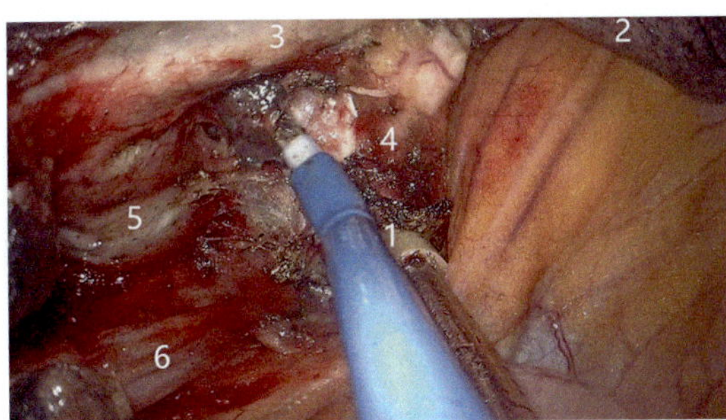

Fig. 4.13 1—Opening of left superior lobar bronchus, 2—inferior lobe of left lung, 3—left inferior pulmonary artery, 4—left inferior lobar bronchus, 5—left pulmonary artery, 6—left superior pulmonary vein. Press the left superior lobar bronchial stump forward and continue to dissect lymph node between artery and bronchus

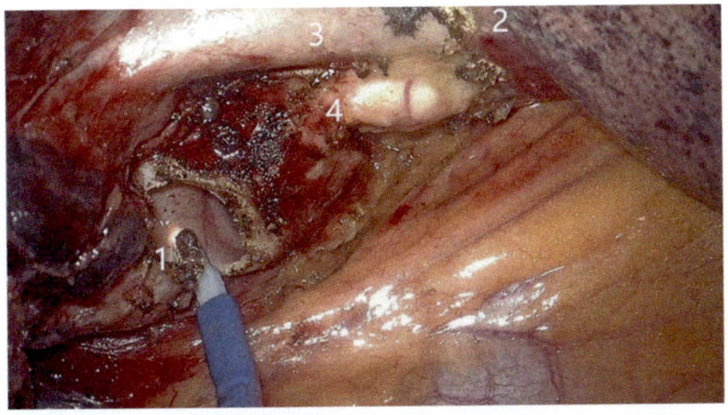

Fig. 4.11 1—Opening of left superior lobar bronchus, 2—inferior lobe of left lung, 3—left inferior pulmonary artery, 4—left inferior lobar bronchus. Cut off left superior lobar bronchus at the opening of left superior lobar bronchus

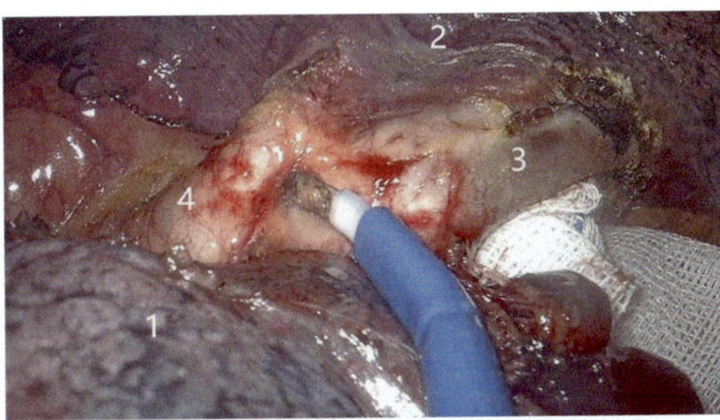

Fig. 4.14 1—Superior lobe of left lung, 2—inferior lobe of left lung, 3—left inferior pulmonary artery, 4—interlobar trunk of left pulmonary artery. Open adventitia of interlobar trunk of left pulmonary artery

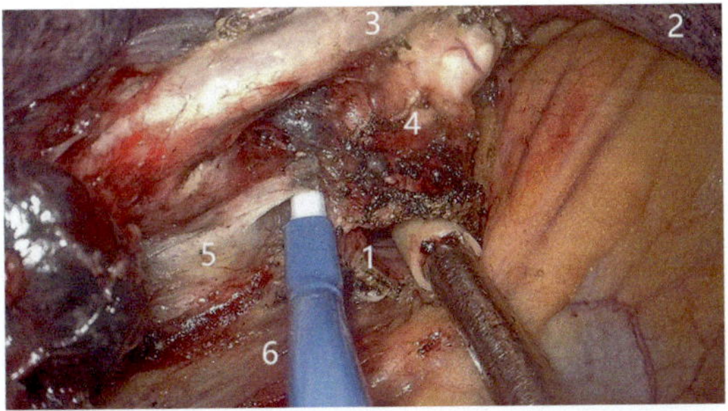

Fig. 4.12 1—Opening of left superior lobar bronchus, 2—inferior lobe of left lung, 3—left inferior pulmonary artery, 4—left inferior lobar bronchus, 5—left pulmonary artery, 6—left superior pulmonary vein. Dissect lymph node along posterior left principal bronchus and anterior left pulmonary artery. Cut off left superior lobar bronchus to reveal the posterior bronchus and anterior pulmonary artery and dissect easily

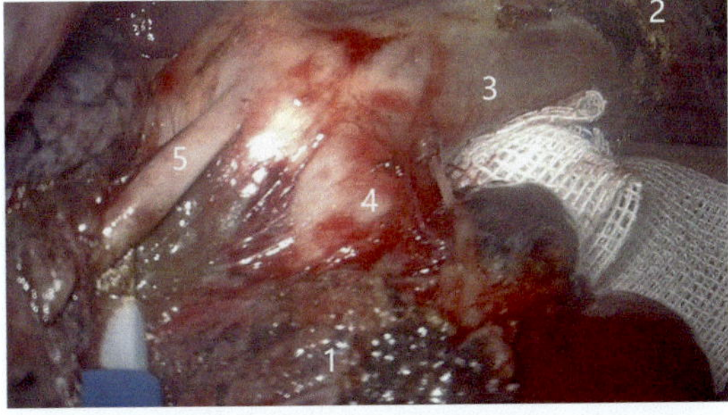

Fig. 4.15 1—Superior lobe of left lung, 2—inferior lobe of left lung, 3—left inferior pulmonary artery, 4—lingual segment artery of superior lobe of left lung, 5—lingual segment artery of superior lobe of left lung. Reveal and dissect lingual segment artery branch of superior lobe of left lung

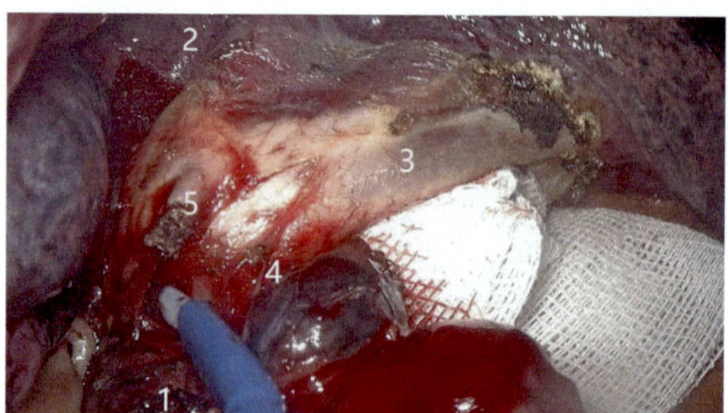

Fig. 4.16 1—Superior lobe of left lung, 2—inferior lobe of left lung, 3—left inferior pulmonary artery, 4—lingual segment artery of superior lobe of left lung, 5—lingual segment artery of superior lobe of left lung. Interrupt the lingual segment artery branch of superior lobe of left lung, for the small pulmonary artery branch; at present, the ultrasonic knife is used to interrupt it. We tried to use the electrotome to interrupt, and the effect is also more satisfactory. Pay attention to the fact that interruption needs enough length

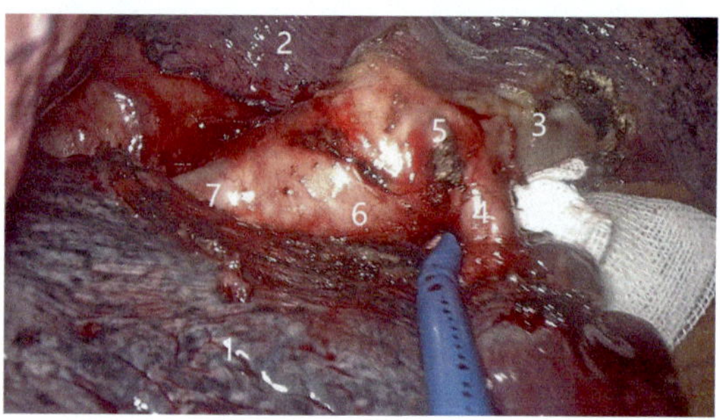

Fig. 4.17 1—Superior lobe of left lung, 2—inferior lobe of left lung, 3—left inferior pulmonary artery, 4—lingual segment artery of superior lobe of left lung, 5—lingual segment artery stump of superior lobe of left lung, 6—interlobar trunk of left pulmonary artery, 7—superior lobe apicoposterior segment artery of left lung. Dissect lingual segment artery of superior lobe of left lung

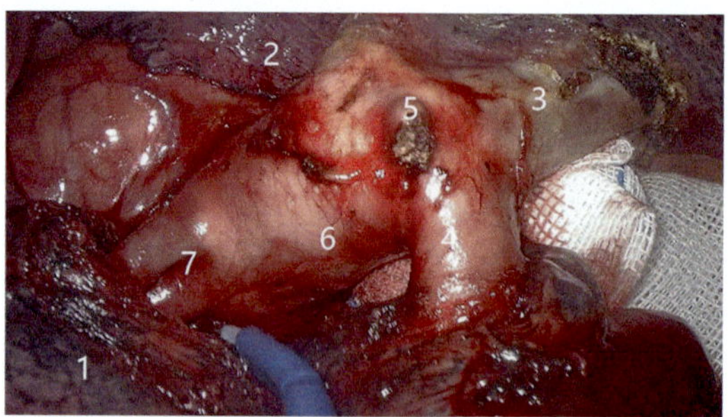

Fig. 4.18 1—Superior lobe of left lung, 2—inferior lobe of left lung, 3—left inferior pulmonary artery, 4—lingual segment artery of superior lobe of left lung, 5—lingual segment artery stump of superior lobe of left lung, 6—interlobar trunk of left pulmonary artery, 7—superior lobe apicoposterior segment artery of left lung. Reveal superior lobe apicoposterior segment artery of left lung

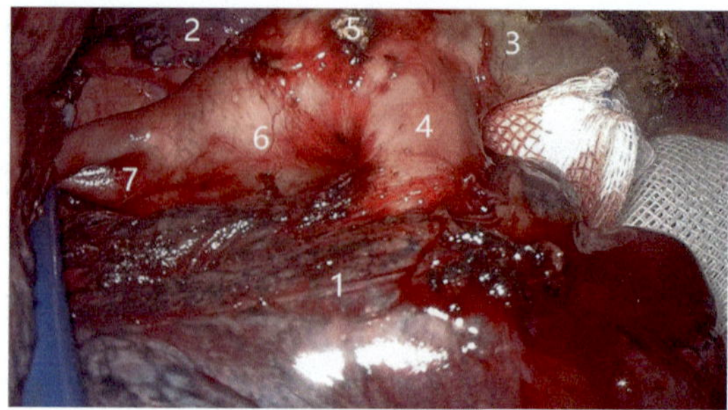

Fig. 4.19 1—Superior lobe of left lung, 2—inferior lobe of left lung, 3—left inferior pulmonary artery, 4—lingual segment artery of superior lobe of left lung, 5—lingual segment artery stump of superior lobe of left lung, 6—interlobar trunk of left pulmonary artery, 7—superior lobe apicoposterior segment artery of left lung. Dissect superior lobe apicoposterior segment artery of left lung and interrupt with GIA

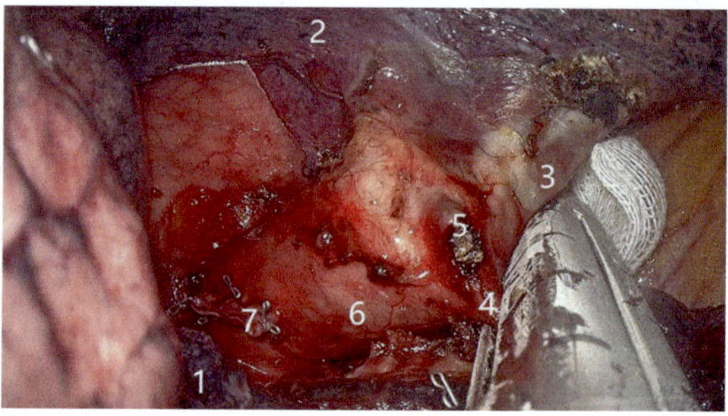

Fig. 4.20 1—Superior lobe of left lung, 2—inferior lobe of left lung, 3—left inferior pulmonary artery, 4—lingual segment artery of superior lobe of left lung, 5—lingual segment artery stump of superior lobe of left lung, 6—interlobar trunk of left pulmonary artery, 7—superior lobe apicoposterior segment artery stump of left lung. Interrupt lingual segment artery of superior lobe of left lung with GIA

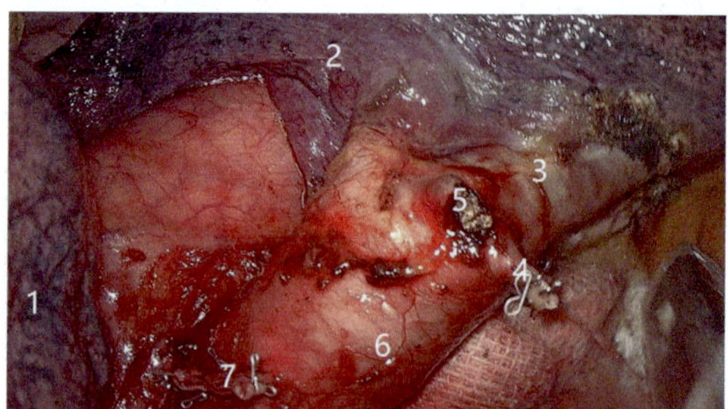

Fig. 4.21 1—Superior lobe of left lung, 2—inferior lobe of left lung, 3—left inferior pulmonary artery, 4—lingual segment artery stump of superior lobe of left lung, 5—lingual segment artery stump of superior lobe of left lung, 6—interlobar trunk of left pulmonary artery, 7—superior lobe apicoposterior segment artery stump of left lung. Showing the interrupted lingual segment artery of superior lobe of left lung and lobe apicoposterior segment artery of left lung

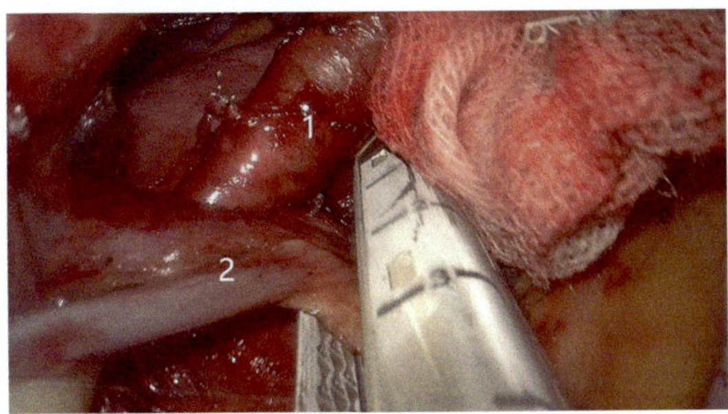

Fig. 4.22 1—Interlobar trunk of left pulmonary artery, 2—left superior pulmonary vein. Dissect left superior pulmonary vein and interrupt with GIA

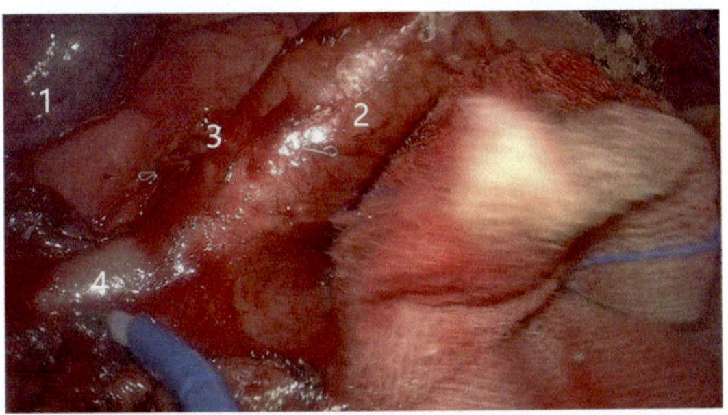

Fig. 4.23 1—Superior lobe of left lung, 2—interlobar trunk of left pulmonary artery, 3—superior lobe apicoposterior segment artery stump of left lung, 4—anterior segment artery of superior lobe of left lung. Reveal anterior segment artery of superior lobe of left lung

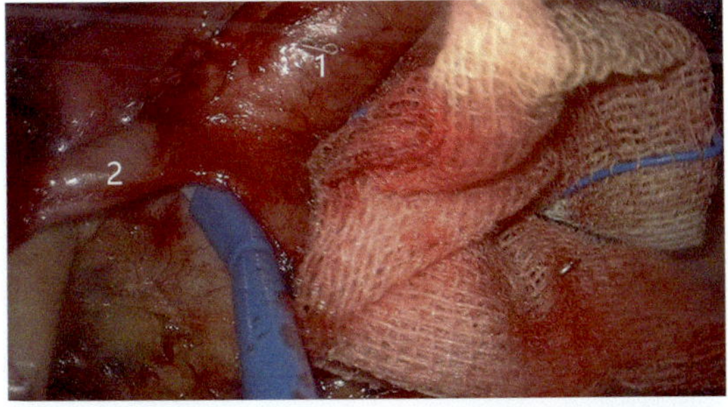

Fig. 4.24 1—Interlobar trunk of left pulmonary artery, 2—anterior segment artery of superior lobe of left lung. Dissect anterior segment artery of superior lobe of left lung and interrupt with GIA

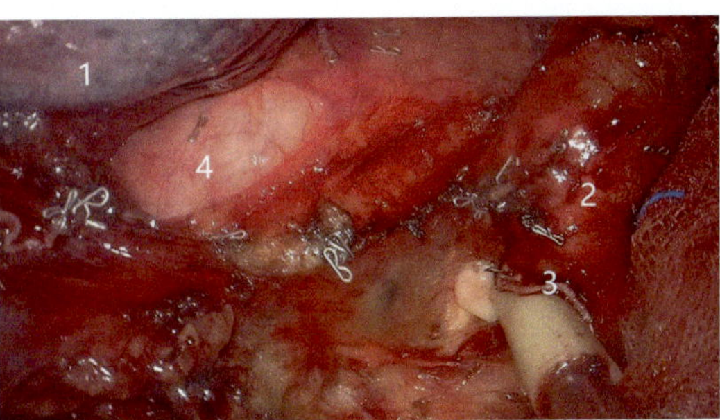

Fig. 4.25 1—Superior lobe of left lung, 2—interlobar trunk of left pulmonary artery, 3—anterior segment artery stump of superior lobe of left lung, 4—descending aorta. Press the pulmonary artery forward and dissect lymph node behind pulmonary artery

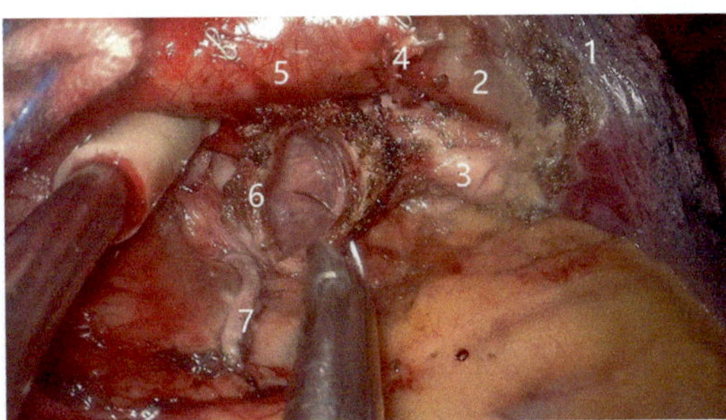

Fig. 4.26 1—Inferior lobe of left lung, 2—left inferior pulmonary artery, 3—left inferior lobar bronchus, 4—lingual segment artery stump of superior lobe of left lung, 5—interlobar trunk of left pulmonary artery, 6—left superior lobar bronchial stump, 7—left superior pulmonary vein stump. Take continuous suture of left superior lobar bronchial stump at the opening of left superior lobar bronchus

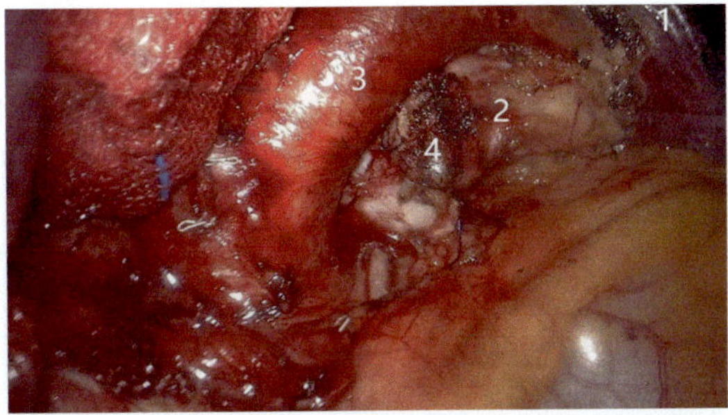

Fig. 4.27 1—Inferior lobe of left lung, 2—left inferior lobar bronchus, 3—interlobar trunk of left pulmonary artery, 4—left superior lobar bronchial stump. Suture is finished

Surgical characteristics: The third intercostal approach is located above the upper lobar bronchi and lingual artery at the level of the interlobar fissure, and its direction of operation is bottom-up separation. After bronchi disconnection, blood vessels can be fully dissociated and extended, providing sufficient space for GIA use. The direction is top-down and anterior-to-backward. This is different from the conventional approach and direction of the fourth and fifth intercostal incisions (Figs. 4.28, 4.29, 4.30, 4.31, 4.32, 4.33, 4.34, 4.35, 4.36, 4.37, 4.38, 4.39, 4.40, 4.41, 4.42, 4.43, 4.44, 4.45, 4.46, 4.47, 4.48, 4.49, 4.50, 4.51, 4.52, 4.53, 4.54, 4.55, 4.56, 4.57, 4.58, 4.59, 4.60, 4.61, 4.62, 4.63, 4.64, and 4.65).

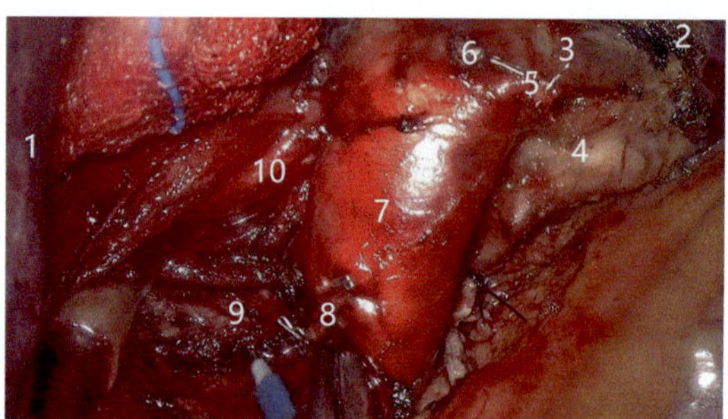

Fig. 4.28 1—Superior lobe of left lung, 2—inferior lobe of left lung, 3—left inferior pulmonary artery, 4—left inferior lobar bronchus, 5—lingual segment artery stump of superior lobe of left lung, 6—lingual segment artery stump of superior lobe of left lung, 7—interlobar trunk of left pulmonary artery, 8—anterior segment artery stump of superior lobe of left lung, 9—trachea, 10—left vagus. Press the pulmonary artery downward and dissect the lymph node above the pulmonary artery to reveal trachea

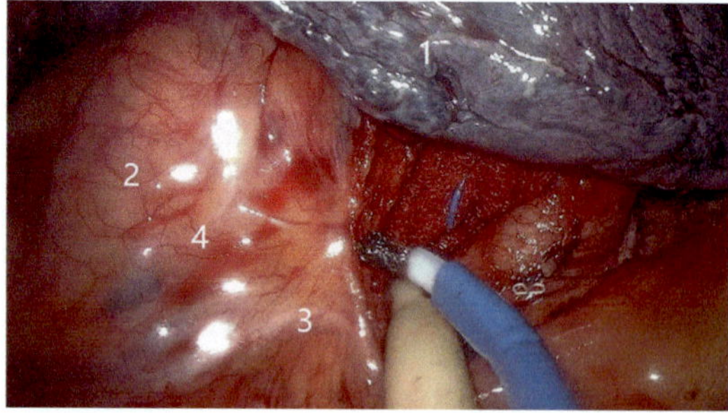

Fig. 4.29 1—Superior lobe of left lung, 2—aortic arch, 3—phrenic nerve, 4—vagus. Open the mediastinum pleura between phrenic nerve and vagus

Summary: The upper lobe lobectomy of the left lung is the more difficult procedure in thoracoscopic lobectomy, and the choice of incision varies according to each individual's custom; we are accustomed to operating through the third

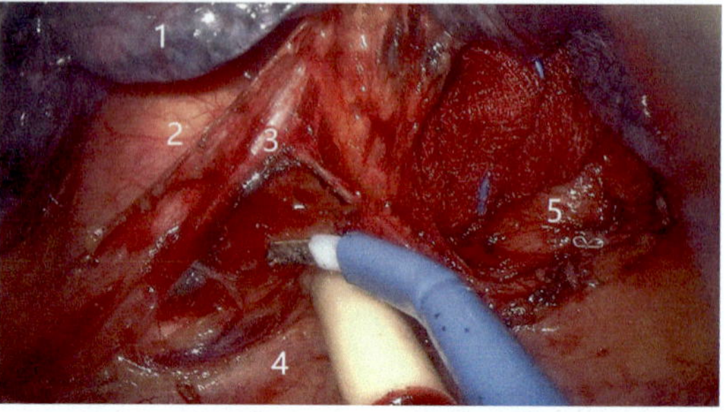

Fig. 4.30 1—Superior lobe of left lung, 2—aortic arch, 3—vagus, 4—phrenic nerve, 5—pulmonary artery. Dissect the lymph node along the anterior vagus downward

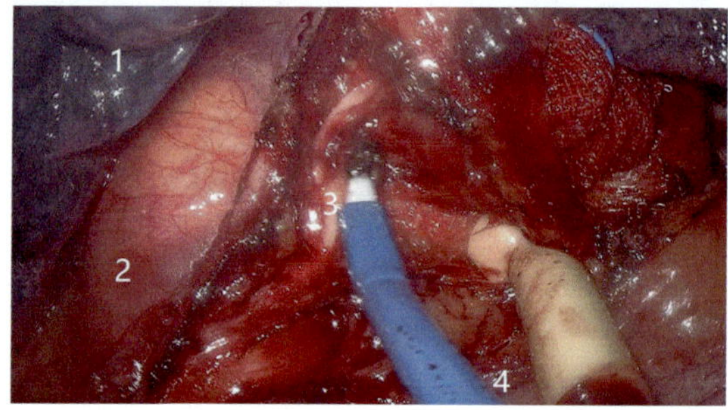

Fig. 4.31 1—Superior lobe of left lung, 2—aortic arch, 3—vagus, 4—phrenic nerve. Dissect the lymph node behind hilum along vagus downward

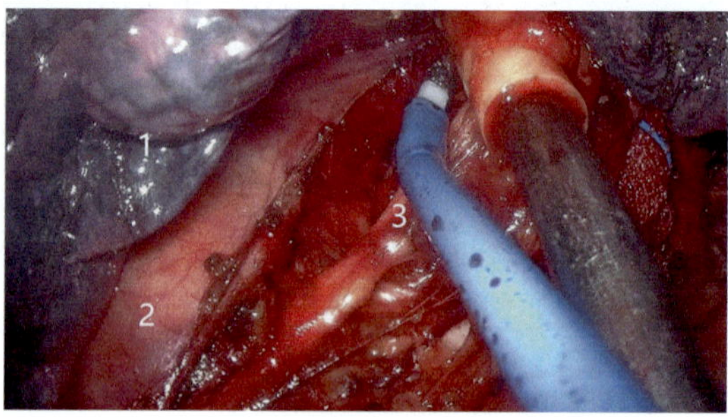

Fig. 4.32 1—Superior lobe of left lung, 2—aortic arch, 3—vagus. Dissect the lymph node in front of descending aorta along vagus

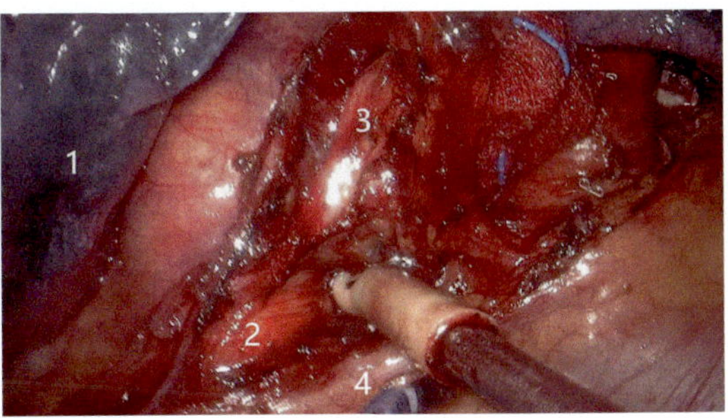

Fig. 4.33 1—Superior lobe of left lung, 2—aortic arch, 3—vagus, 4—phrenic nerve. Dissect the lymph node along the surface of phrenic nerve

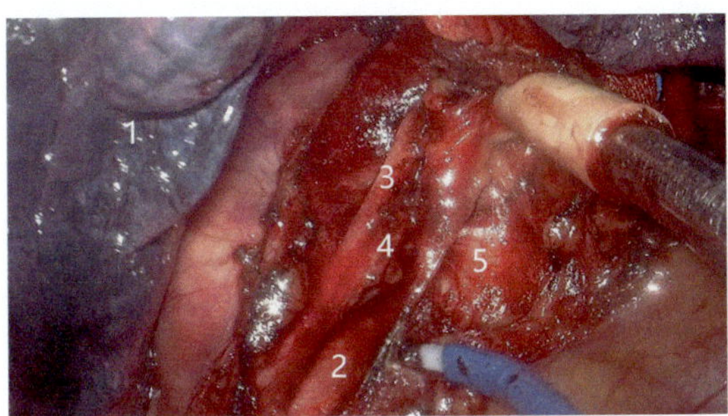

Fig. 4.34 1—Superior lobe of left lung, 2—aortic arch, 3—vagus, 4—beginning of recurrent laryngeal nerve, 5—arterial ligament. Dissect the lymph node along phrenic nerve backward to reveal arterial ligament and beginning of recurrent laryngeal nerve

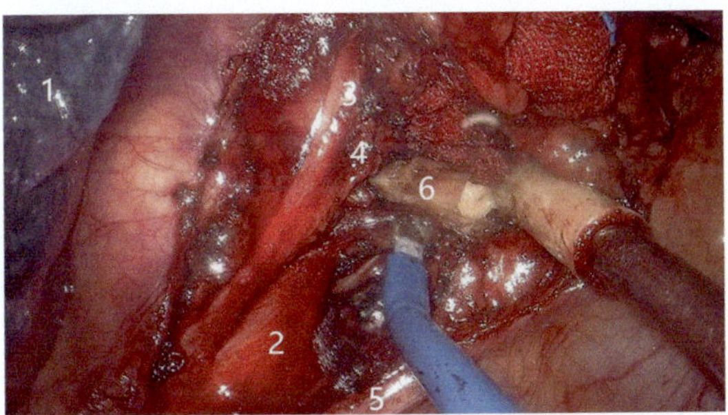

Fig. 4.35 1—Superior lobe of left lung, 2—aortic arch, 3—vagus, 4—beginning of recurrent laryngeal nerve, 5—phrenic nerve, 6—arterial ligament

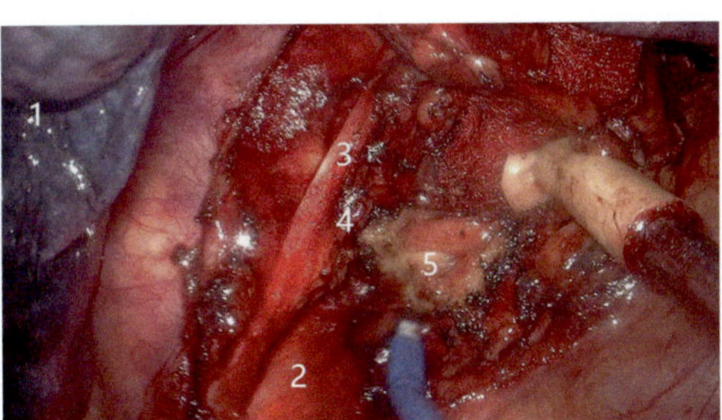

Fig. 4.36 1—Superior lobe of left lung, 2—aortic arch, 3—vagus, 4—beginning of recurrent laryngeal nerve, 5—arterial ligament. Interrupt arterial ligament

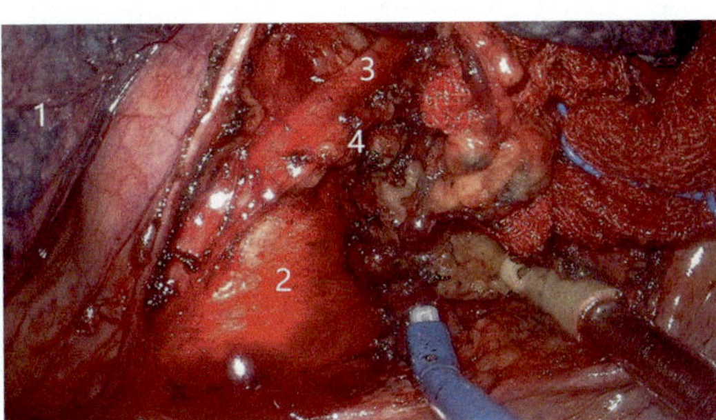

Fig. 4.37 1—Superior lobe of left lung, 2—aortic arch, 3—vagus, 4—beginning of recurrent laryngeal nerve. Dissect the lymph node behind arterial ligament along inferior aorta

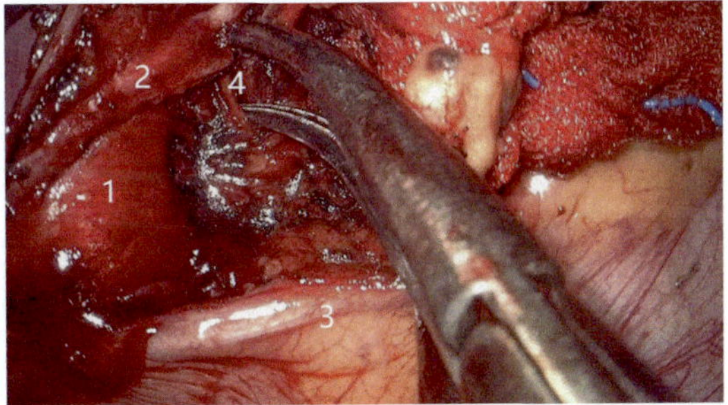

Fig. 4.38 1—Aortic arch, 2—vagus, 3—phrenic nerve, 4—recurrent laryngeal nerve. Reveal recurrent laryngeal nerve

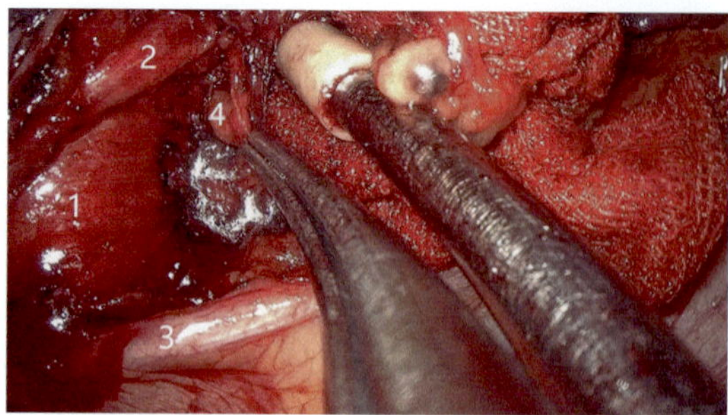

Fig. 4.39 1—Aortic arch, 2—vagus, 3—phrenic nerve, 4—recurrent laryngeal nerve. Dissect the lymph node along recurrent laryngeal nerve upward and backward

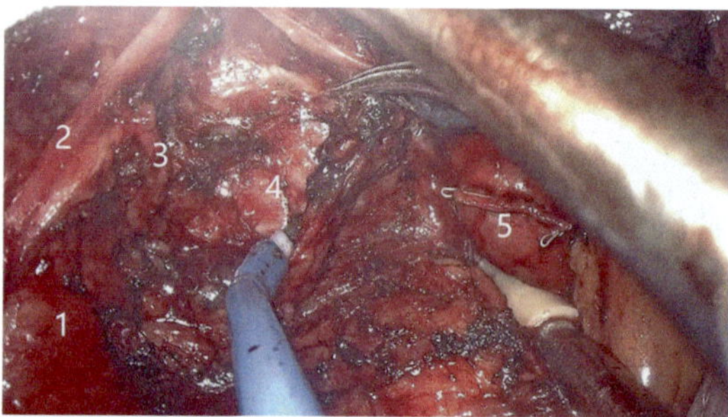

Fig. 4.40 1—Aortic arch, 2—vagus, 3—recurrent laryngeal nerve, 4—trachea, 5—left pulmonary artery. Dissect the lymph node along inferior recurrent laryngeal nerve downward

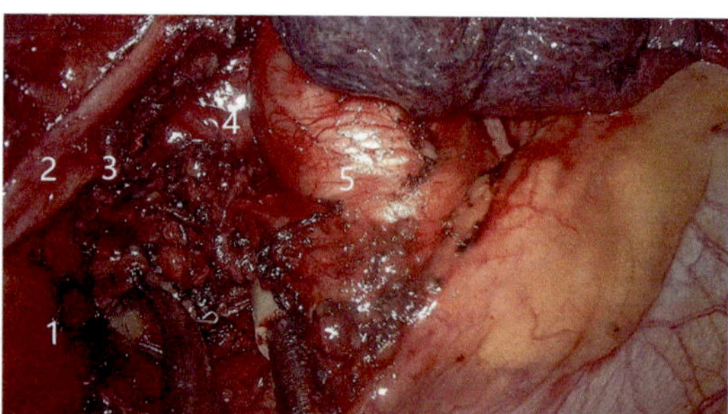

Fig. 4.41 1—Aortic arch, 2—vagus, 3—recurrent laryngeal nerve, 4—trachea, 5—left pulmonary artery. Dissect the lymph node at the inferior of aortic arch along posterior pericardium upward and backward

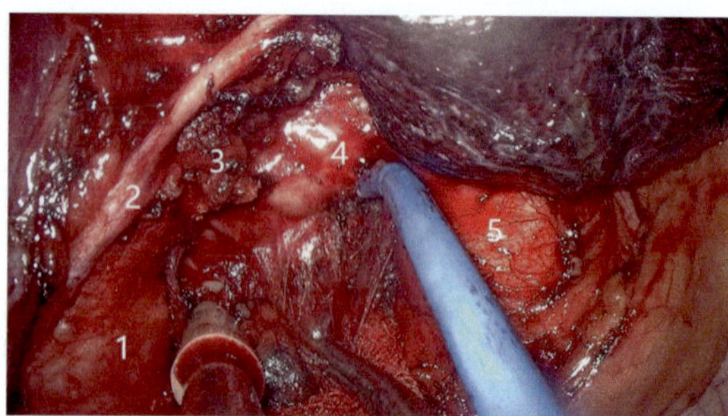

Fig. 4.42 1—Aortic arch, 2—vagus, 3—recurrent laryngeal nerve, 4—trachea, 5—left pulmonary artery. Dissect the lymph node along anterior trachea forward

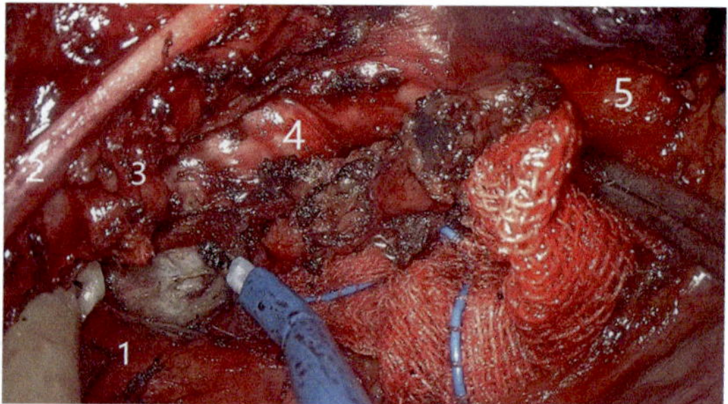

Fig. 4.43 1—Aortic arch, 2—vagus, 3—recurrent laryngeal nerve, 4—trachea, 5—left pulmonary artery. Dissect the lymph node along anterior trachea downward at the posterior of aortic arch

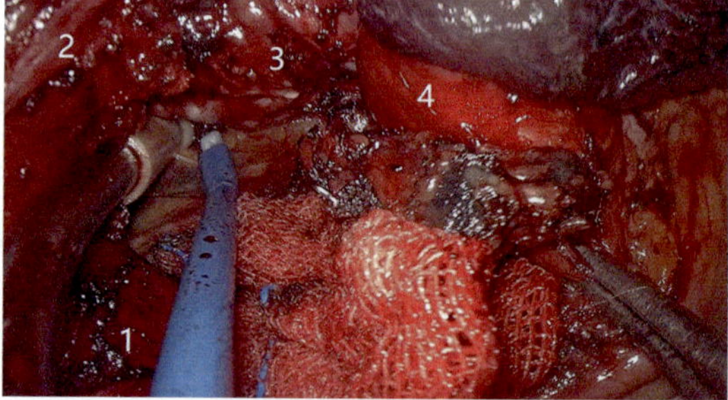

Fig. 4.44 1—Aortic arch, 2—vagus, 3—trachea, 4—left pulmonary artery. Dissect the lymph node along posterior trachea downward

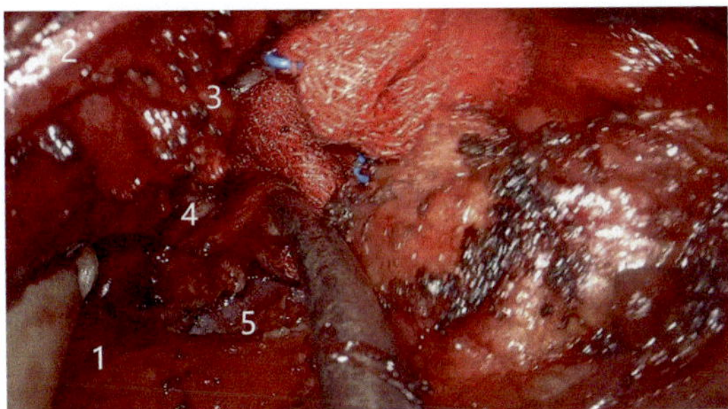

Fig. 4.45 1—Aortic arch, 2—vagus, 3—recurrent laryngeal nerve, 4—trachea, 5—superior vena cava. Reveal superior vena cava, dissect the lymph node along the surface of superior vena cava backward

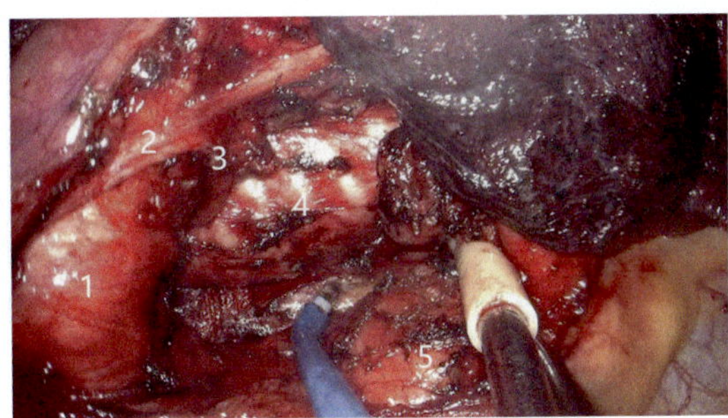

Fig. 4.48 1—Aortic arch, 2—vagus, 3—recurrent laryngeal nerve, 4—trachea, 5—left pulmonary artery. Dissect the lymph node along anterior trachea to superior left principal bronchus

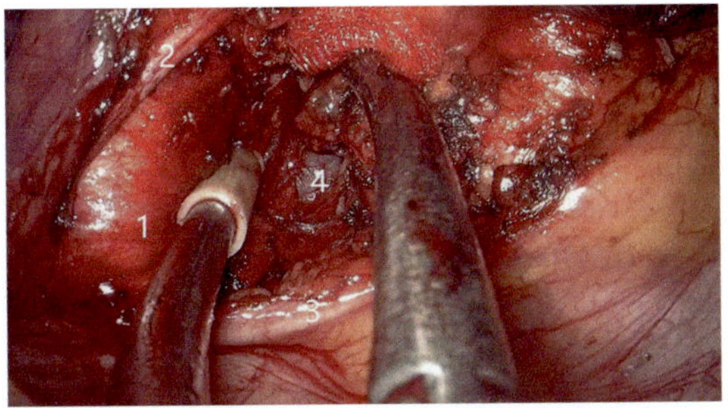

Fig. 4.46 1—Aortic arch, 2—vagus, 3—phrenic nerve, 4—superior vena cava. Dissect the lymph node along superior vena cava downward

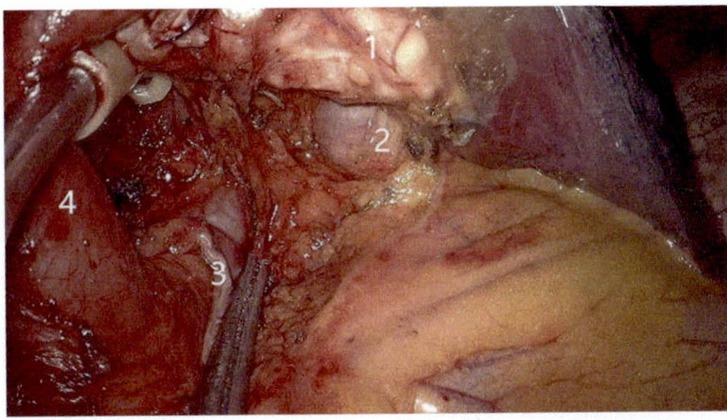

Fig. 4.49 1—Left inferior lobar bronchus, 2—left inferior pulmonary vein, 3—left superior pulmonary vein stump, 4—left pulmonary artery. Dissect the lymph node along posterior pericardium backward and downward

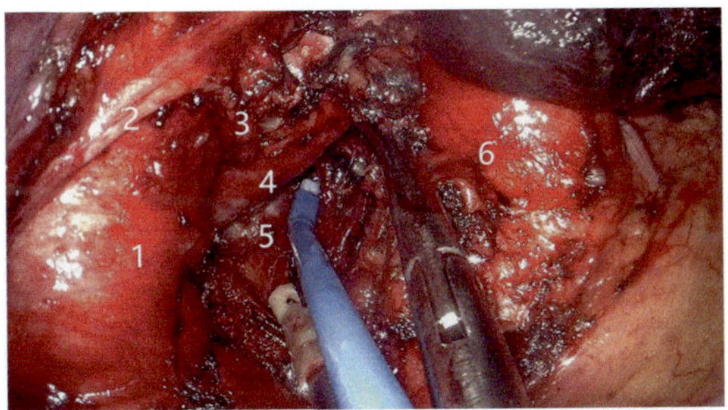

Fig. 4.47 1—Aortic arch, 2—vagus, 3—recurrent laryngeal nerve, 4—trachea, 5—arch of azygos vein, 6—left pulmonary artery. Reveal arch of azygos vein, dissect the lymph node along the surface of arch of azygos vein downward

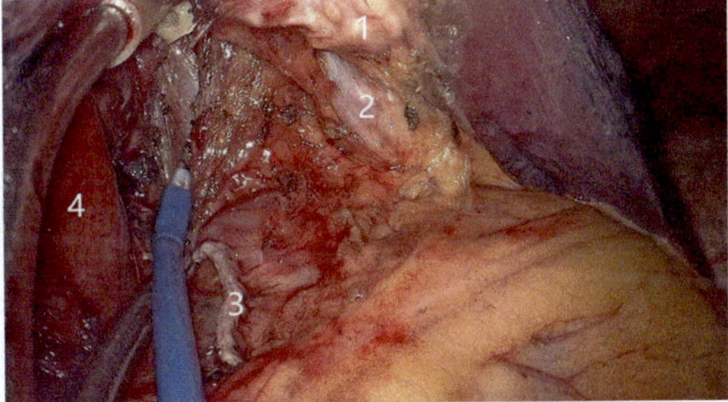

Fig. 4.50 1—Left inferior lobar bronchus, 2—left inferior pulmonary vein, 3—left superior pulmonary vein stump, 4—left pulmonary artery. Dissect the lymph node backward to reveal esophagus

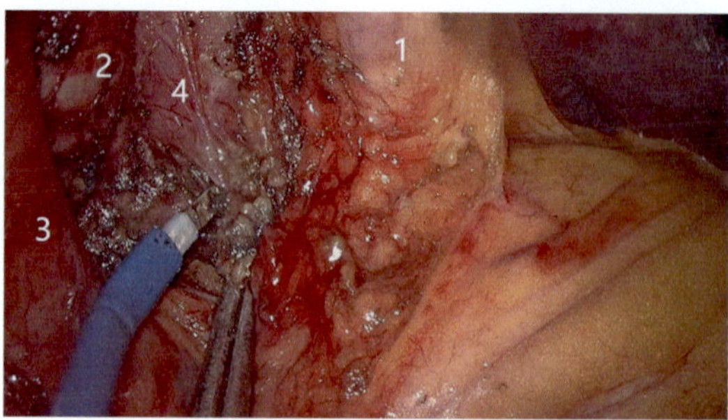

Fig. 4.51 1—Left inferior pulmonary vein, 2—left principal bronchus, 3—left pulmonary artery, 4—esophagus. Dissect the lymph node along the surface of esophagus forward

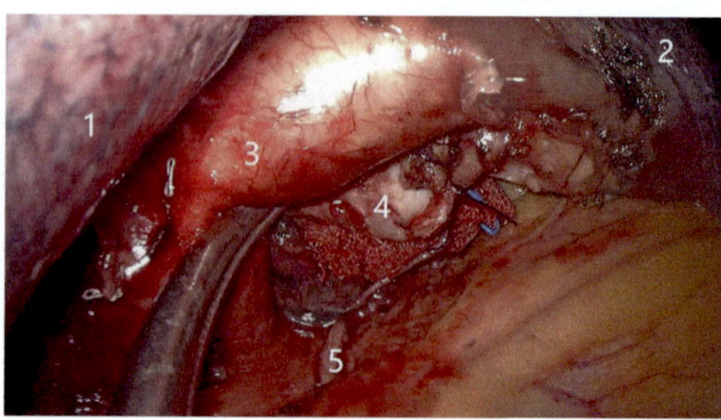

Fig. 4.54 1—Superior lobe of left lung, 2—inferior lobe of left lung, 3—interlobar trunk of left pulmonary artery, 4—left principal bronchus, 5—left superior pulmonary vein stump. Showing the lymph node dissected along the trachea downward

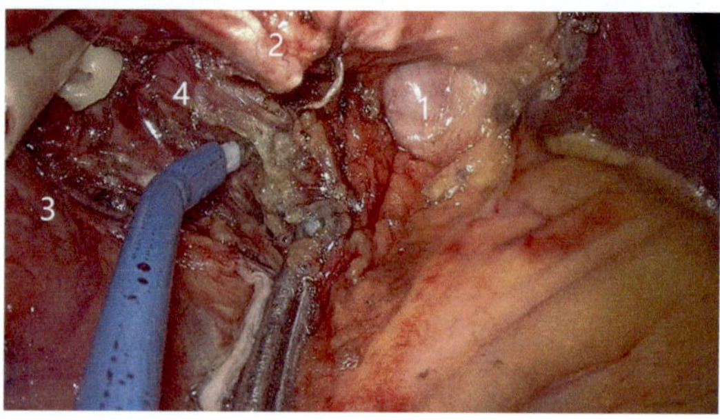

Fig. 4.52 1—Left inferior pulmonary vein, 2—left inferior lobar bronchus, 3—left pulmonary artery, 4—esophagus. Dissect the lymph node along esophagus downward and backward

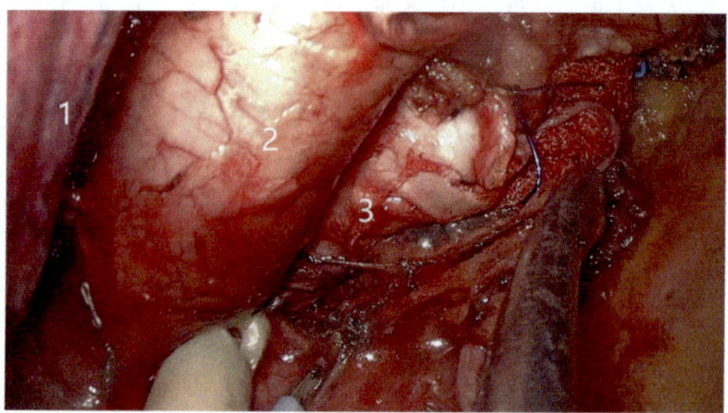

Fig. 4.55 1—Superior lobe of left lung, 2—interlobar trunk of left pulmonary artery, 3—left principal bronchus. Dissect the lymph node along posterior pericardium backward, and resect it with the lymph node dissected along the trachea downward en bloc

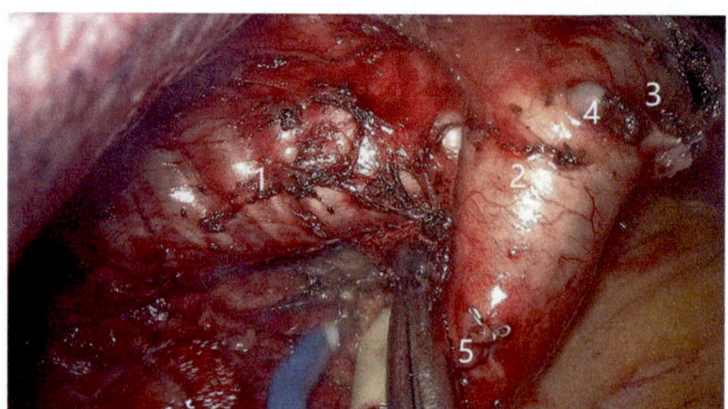

Fig. 4.53 1—Trachea, 2—interlobar trunk of left pulmonary artery, 3—left inferior pulmonary artery, 4—lingual segment artery stump of superior lobe of left lung, 5—superior lobe apicoposterior segment artery stump of left lung. Press the left pulmonary artery forward and downward, dissect the lymph node along anterior trachea across the carina, and the gauze pressed against the carina is visible

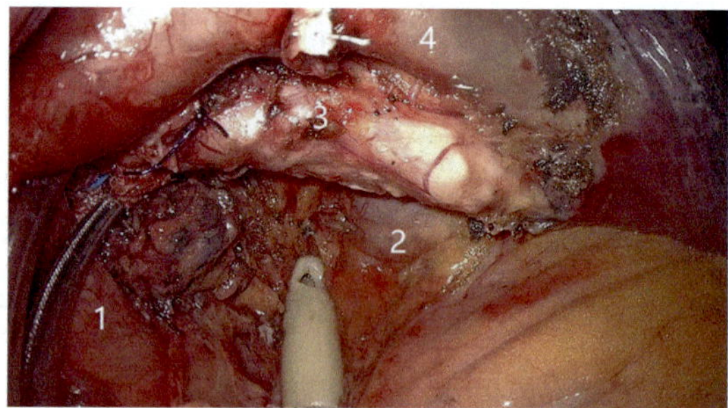

Fig. 4.56 1—Left pulmonary artery, 2—left inferior pulmonary vein, 3—left inferior lobar bronchus, 4—left inferior pulmonary artery. Dissect the lymph node along left inferior pulmonary vein backward

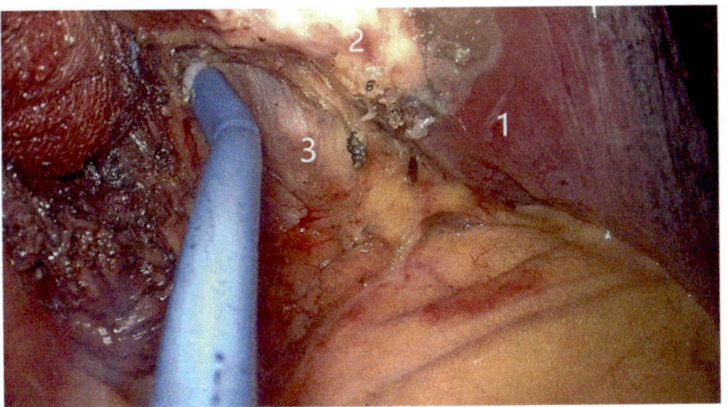

Fig. 4.57 1—Left pulmonary artery, 2—left inferior lobar bronchus, 3—left inferior pulmonary vein. Dissect the lymph node along left inferior pulmonary vein backward and upward to the anterior esophagus

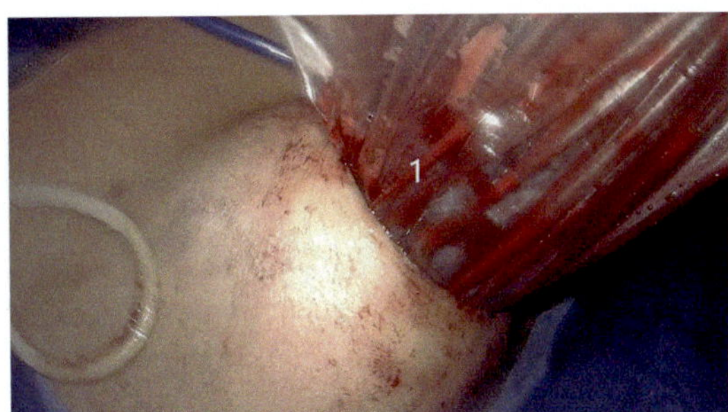

Fig. 4.60 1—Specimen. Take out the specimen

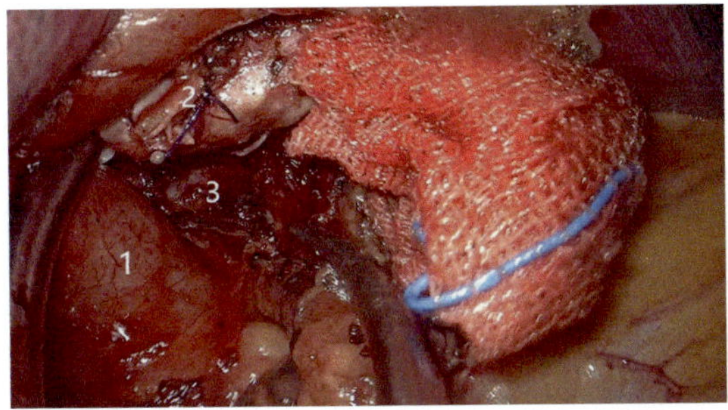

Fig. 4.58 1—Left pulmonary artery, 2—left superior lobar bronchial stump, 3—right principal bronchus. Reveal right principal bronchus and dissect the lymph node along right principal bronchus downward

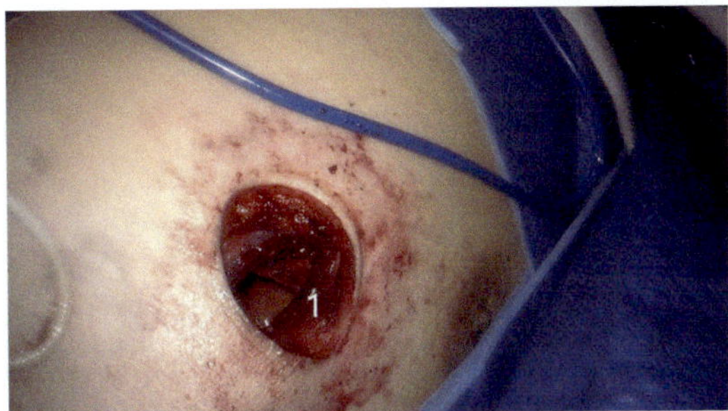

Fig. 4.61 1—Incision. Showing the incision resecting the specimen

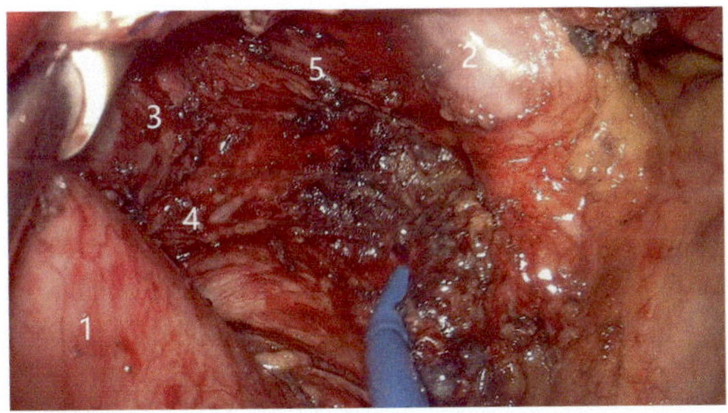

Fig. 4.59 1—Left pulmonary artery, 2—left inferior pulmonary vein, 3—left principal bronchus, 4—right principal bronchus, 5—esophagus. Dissect the lymph node along right principal bronchus downward, and connect to the lymph node dissected along left inferior pulmonary vein, and resect the lymph node en bloc

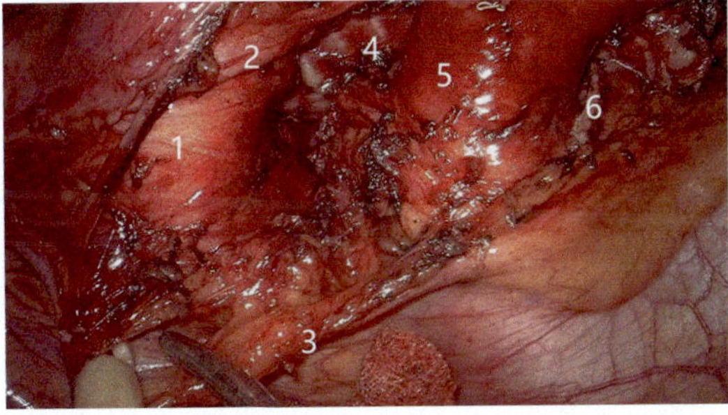

Fig. 4.62 1—Aortic arch, 2—vagus, 3—phrenic nerve, 4—trachea, 5—left pulmonary artery, 6—left superior pulmonary vein stump. Dissect the lymph node along phrenic nerve to superior aortic arch forward

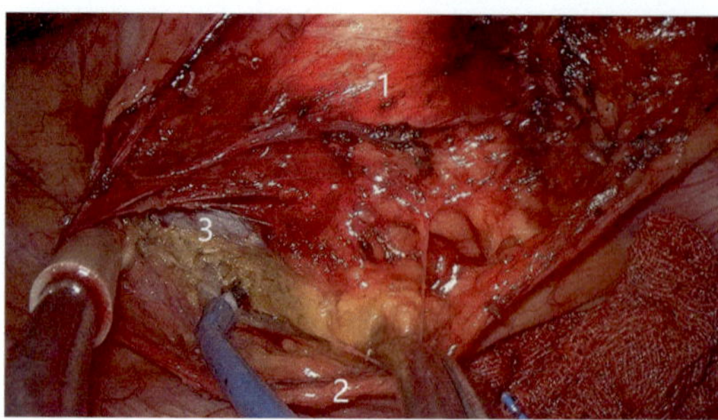

Fig. 4.63 1—Aortic arch, 2—phrenic nerve, 3—left innominate vein. Reveal the left innominate vein, dissect the lymph node along left innominate vein downward

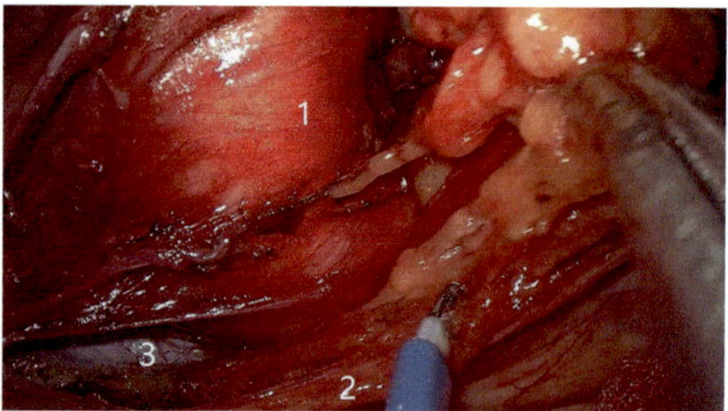

Fig. 4.64 1—Aortic arch, 2—phrenic nerve, 3—left innominate vein. Finish the lymph node dissection along anterior and superior aortic arch

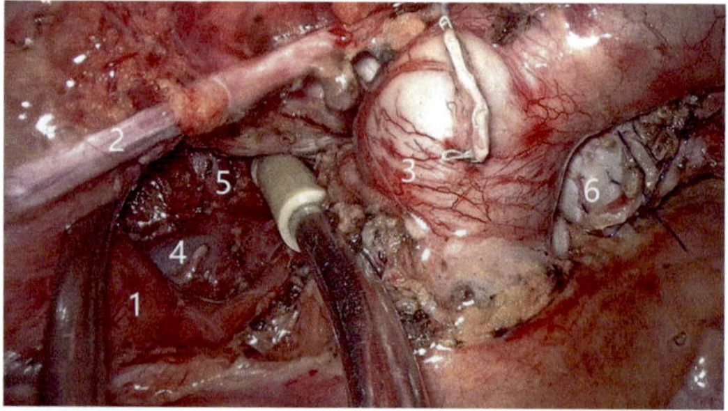

Fig. 4.65 1—Aortic arch, 2—vagus, 3—left pulmonary artery, 4—superior vena cava, 5—trachea, 6—left principal bronchus. Surgery is finished

intercostal incision in the anterior axillary line, which is horizontal above the pulmonary hilum and very convenient for lymph node dissection above the pulmonary hilum and in the pulmonary artery window.

This case demonstrates a complete lymph nodes dissection from below the aortic arch, above the inferior pulmonary vein, posterior to the pulmonary hilum and pericardium, anterior to the esophagus, and including the right group 4 lymph nodes. The dissection starts from the anterior aspect of the pulmonary hilum, and after dissection of the bronchi of the upper lobe of the left lung, it is very favorable to remove the groups of lymph nodes between the upper and lower lobes from the bottom to the top, while the branches of the upper lobe arteries behind the bronchi are fully exposed; after dissection of the branches of the vessels of the upper lobe, the pulmonary arteries are dissociated, which makes the surrounding lymph nodes more fully exposed; the lymph nodes of the pulmonary artery window should be removed with a holistic concept; the area behind the pericardium, behind the aortic arch, and in front of the descending aorta should be considered as a whole, and the vagus nerve should be removed along the vagus nerve from under the aortic arch downward to reveal the recurrent laryngeal nerve, starting from the phrenic nerve and posterior to the pericardium and removing posteriorly, the superior vena cava and recurrent laryngeal nerve can be displayed after dissection of the arterial ligament, upward and downward dissection of lymph nodes around the trachea along the recurrent laryngeal nerve, forward and right separation along the trachea, can display the arch of azygos vein, downward dissection along the arch of azygos vein to the front of the protuberance, complete the pulmonary artery window dissection. The entire lymph tissue in the pulmonary artery window area was removed downward from the gap between the trachea and the pulmonary artery to connect with the protuberance. The lymph nodes in the protuberance area were removed downward, and the lymph nodes were removed upward and backward along the lower pulmonary vein to the lymph nodes in front of the esophagus to complete the whole dissection of the lymph nodes.

5 Excision of the Left Inferior Lobe of Lung

Thoracoscopic left inferior lobectomy is relatively simple in lung lobectomy, and the third intercostal left inferior lobectomy is basically performed above the lower lobe of the left lung, with slightly different spatial structure (Figs. 5.1, 5.2, 5.3, 5.4, 5.5, 5.6, 5.7, 5.8, 5.9, 5.10, 5.11, 5.12, 5.13, 5.14, 5.15, 5.16, 5.17, 5.18, 5.19, 5.20, 5.21, 5.22, 5.23, 5.24, 5.25, 5.26, 5.27, 5.28, 5.29, 5.30, 5.31, 5.32, 5.33, and 5.34).

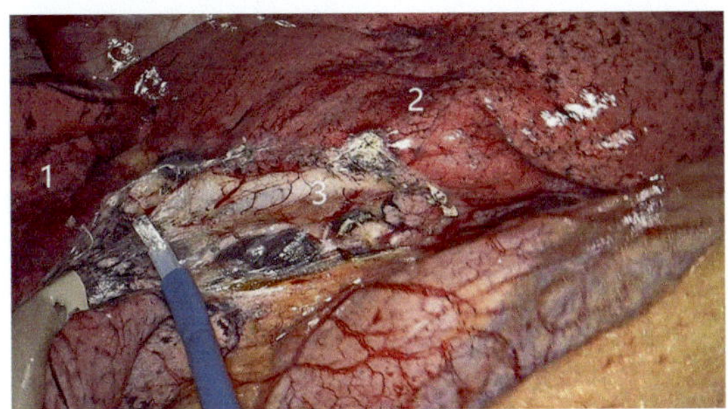

Fig. 5.1 1—Upper lobe of left lung, 2—lower lobe of left lung, 3—basilar artery of left lower lobe of left lung. Open the interlobar fissure and expose the interlobar vessels

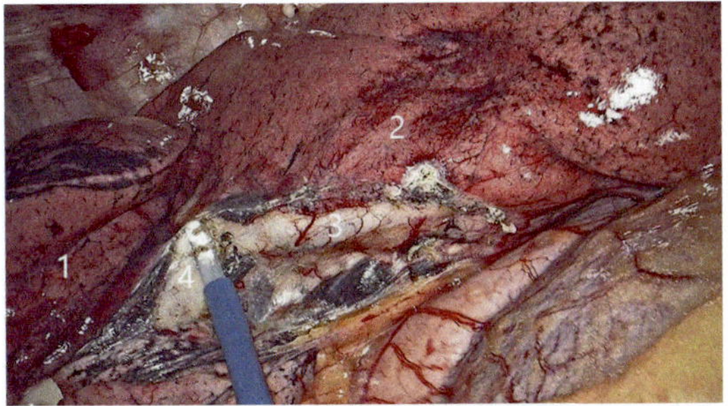

Fig. 5.2 1—Upper lobe of left lung, 2—lower lobe of left lung, 3—basal segment artery of lower lobe of left lung, 4—lingual segment artery of upper lobe of left lung. Open the interlobar vasculature

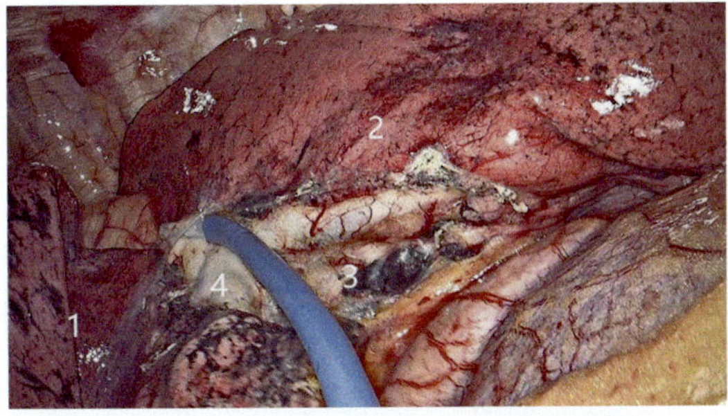

Fig. 5.3 1—Upper lobe of the left lung, 2—lower lobe of the left lung, 3—bronchus of the lower lobe of the left lung, 4—lingual artery of the upper lobe of the left lung. It travels backward along the interlobar vessels

J. Li, Z. Long, *Atlas of Thoracoscopic Lobectomy with Bronchoplasty*,
https://doi.org/10.1007/978-981-99-5150-5_5

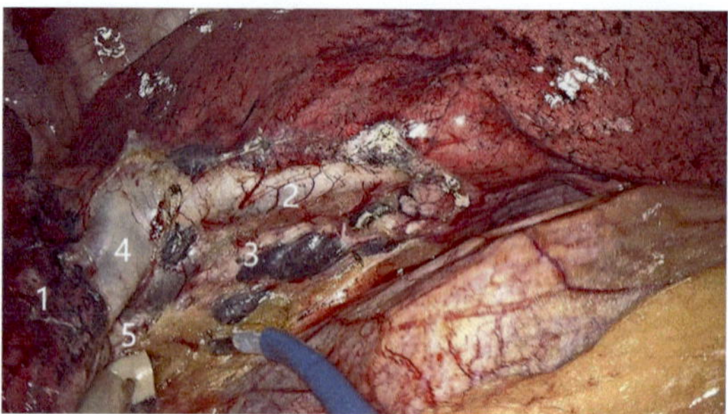

Fig. 5.4 1—Upper lobe of the left lung, 2—basal segment artery of the lower lobe of the left lung, 3—bronchi of the lower lobe of the left lung, 4—artery of the upper lobe of the left lung, 5—bronchi of the upper lobe of the left lung. Lymph nodes were swept down the superior pulmonary vein

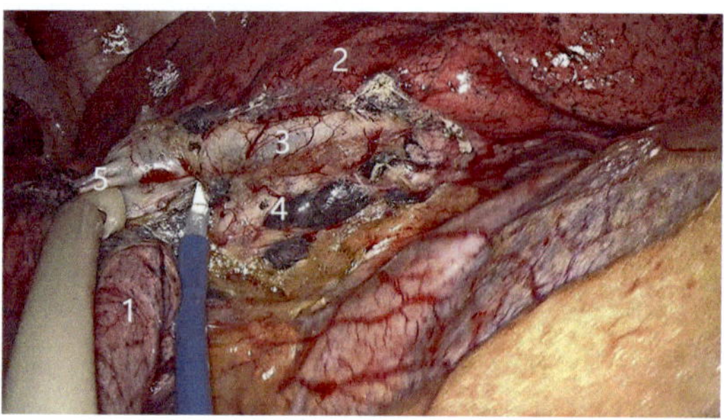

Fig. 5.5 1—Upper lobe of left lung, 2—lower lobe of left lung, 3—basal segment artery of lower lobe of left lung, 4—bronchus of lower lobe of left lung, 5—lingual segment artery of upper lobe of left lung. Sweep down the anterior direction of the basal artery of the left inferior lobe of the left lung, below the lingual artery of the left superior lobe

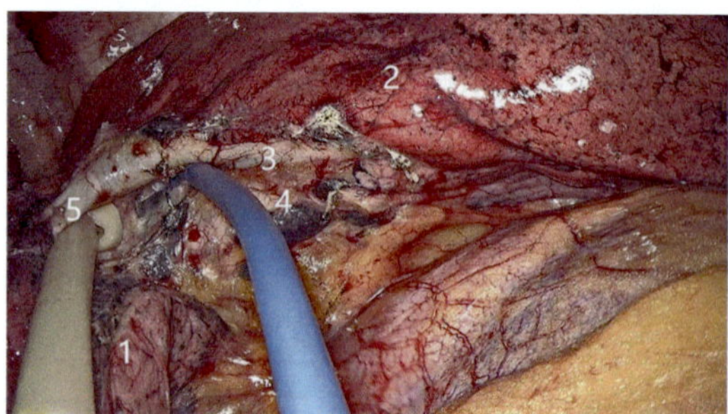

Fig. 5.6 1—Upper lobe of left lung, 2—lower lobe of left lung, 3—basal segment artery of lower lobe of left lung, 4—bronchus of lower lobe of left lung, 5—lingual segment artery of upper lobe of left lung. Lymph nodes posterior to the lower basal artery of the left inferior lobe were cleared

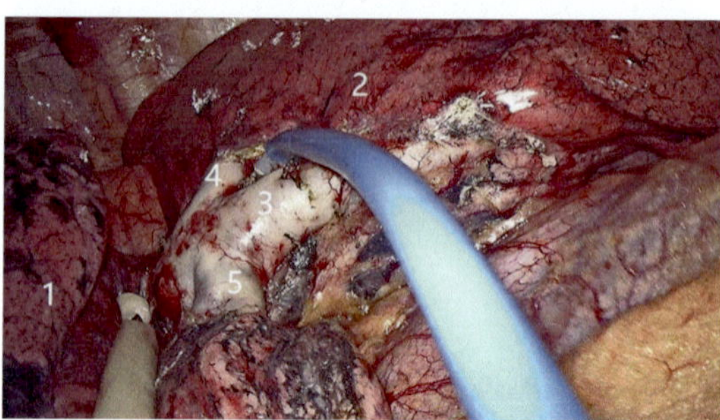

Fig. 5.7 1—Upper lobe of left lung, 2—lower lobe of left lung, 3—basal segment artery of lower lobe of left lung, 4—dorsal segment artery of lower lobe of left lung, 5—lingual segment artery of upper lobe of left lung. The left inferior lobe of the left lung is left behind the basal artery to reveal the left inferior lobe of the left dorsal artery

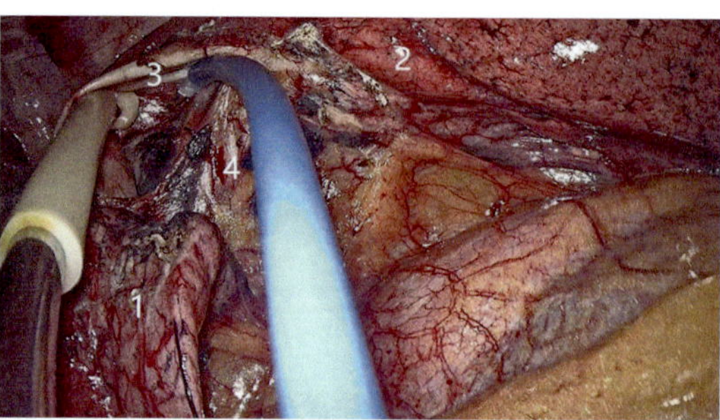

Fig. 5.8 1—Upper lobe of left lung, 2—lower lobe of left lung, 3—lower lobe artery of left lung, 4—bronchus of left lower lobe of left lung. Lymph nodes behind the dorsal artery of the left inferior lobe of the lung were cleared and the dorsal artery was dissociated

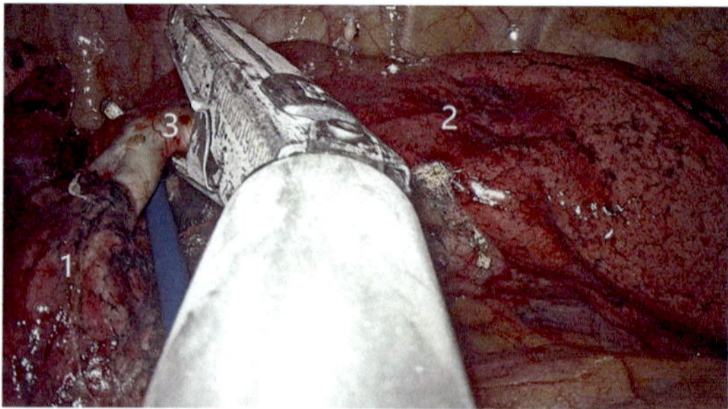

Fig. 5.9 1—Upper lobe of left lung, 2—lower lobe of left lung, 3—lower lobe of left lung artery. GIA was used at the left inferior pulmonary artery opening

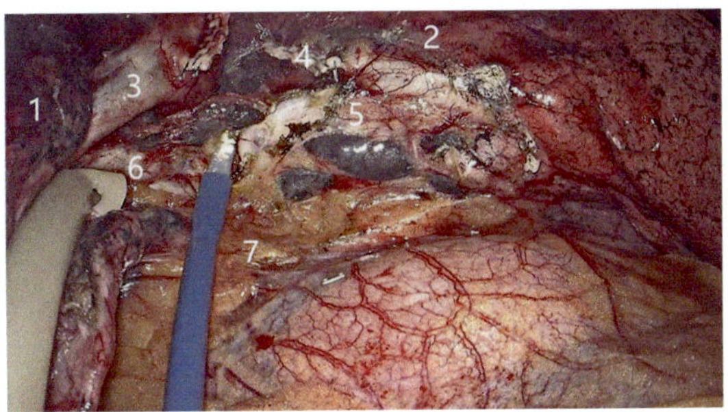

Fig. 5.10 1—Upper lobe of the left lung, 2—lower lobe of the left lung, 3—arteries of the upper lobe of the left lung, 4—stump of the lower lobe artery of the left lung, 5—bronchi of the lower lobe of the left lung, 6—bronchi of the upper lobe of the left lung, 7—veins of the upper lobe of the left lung. Sweep down the left superior lobar bronchus behind the left superior lobar vein

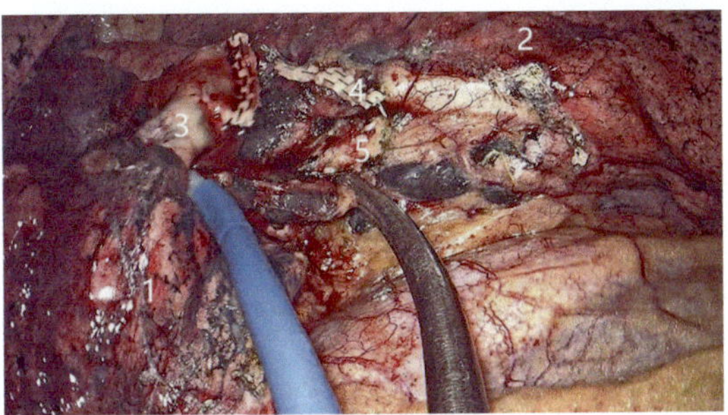

Fig. 5.11 1—Upper lobe of the left lung, 2—lower lobe of the left lung, 3—lingual artery of the upper lobe of the left lung, 4—stump of the lower lobe artery of the left lung, 5—bronchus of the lower lobe of the left lung. Lymph nodes posterior to the lingual artery of the left superior lobe were cleared

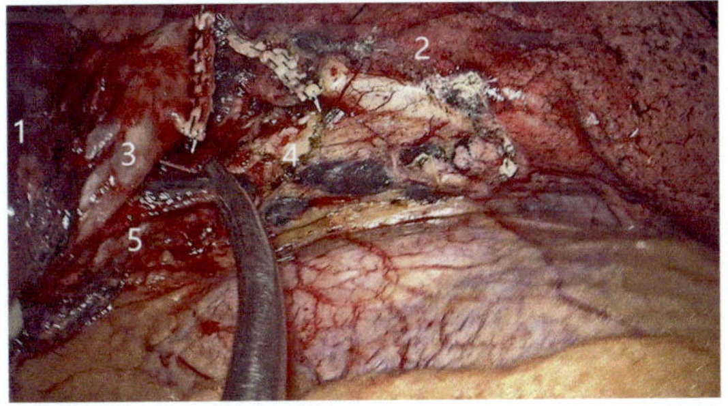

Fig. 5.12 1—Upper lobe of the left lung, 2—lower lobe of the left lung, 3—lingual artery of the upper lobe of the left lung, 4—stump of the lower lobe artery of the left lung, 5—bronchus of the lower lobe of the left lung. Lymph nodes behind the bronchus of the left superior lobar were swept up along the artery of the left superior lobar lobe

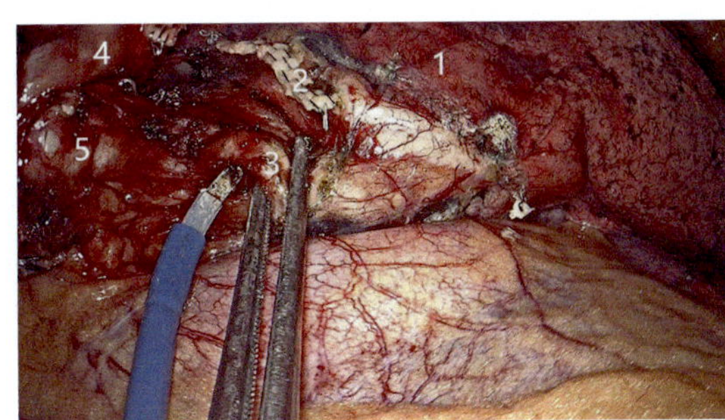

Fig. 5.13 1—Lower lobe of the left lung, 2—stump of the lower lobe artery of the left lung, 3—bronchi of the lower lobe of the left lung, 4—arteries of the upper lobe of the left lung, 5—bronchi of the upper lobe of the left lung. The left inferior lobar bronchus was severed at the opening of the left inferior lobar bronchus

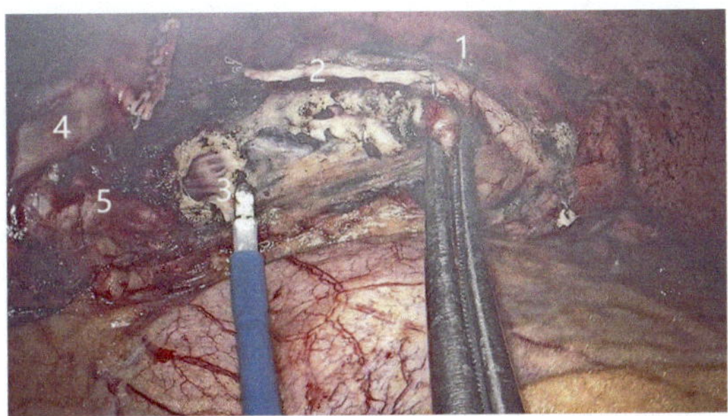

Fig. 5.14 1—Lower lobe of the left lung, 2—lower lobe artery stump of the left lung, 3—bronchial stump of the lower lobe of the left lung, 4—lingual artery of the upper lobe of the left lung, 5—upper lobe bronchi of the left lung. Lymph nodes below and behind the bronchial stump of the left inferior lobe were cleared

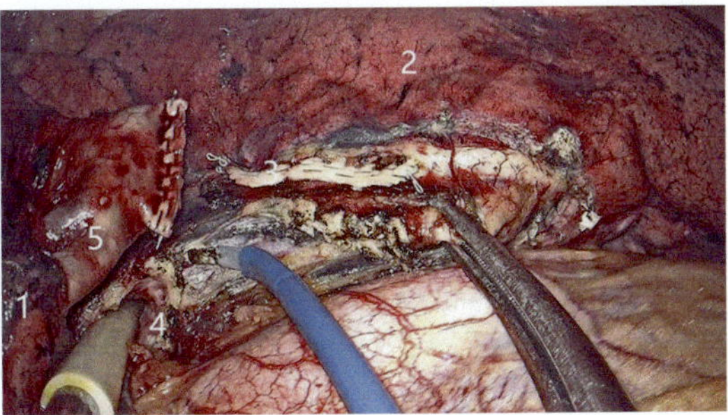

Fig. 5.15 1—Upper lobe of the left lung, 2—lower lobe of the left lung, 3—stump of the lower lobe artery of the left lung, 4—stump of the bronchus of the lower lobe of the left lung, 5—artery of the upper lobe of the left lung. Sweep below the left main bronchus

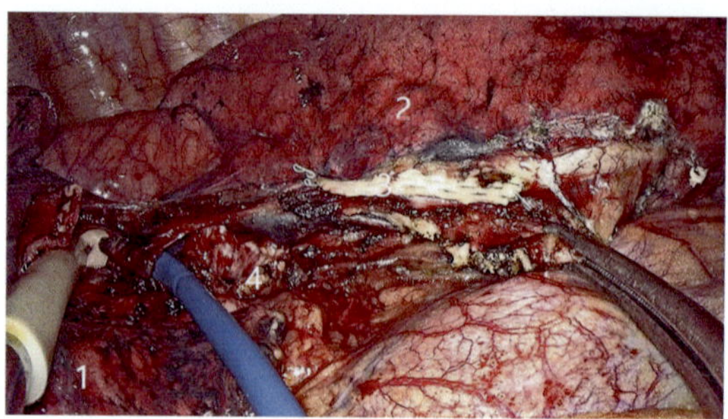

Fig. 5.16 1—Upper lobe of left lung, 2—lower lobe of left lung, 3—lower lobe artery stump of left lung, 4—bronchial stump of left lower lobe of left lung. Lymph nodes posterior to the left superior lobar bronchus were cleared

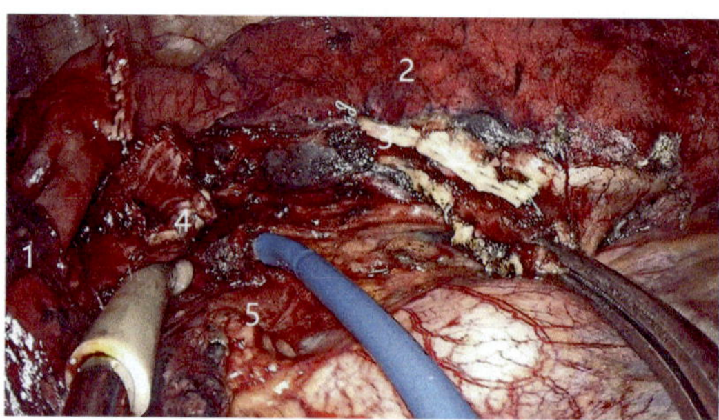

Fig. 5.17 1—Upper lobe of the left lung, 2—lower lobe of the left lung, 3—stump of the lower lobe artery of the left lung, 4—stump of the bronchus of the lower lobe of the left lung, 5—vein of the upper lobe of the left lung. Sweep posteriorly along left superior pulmonary vein and posterior pericardium

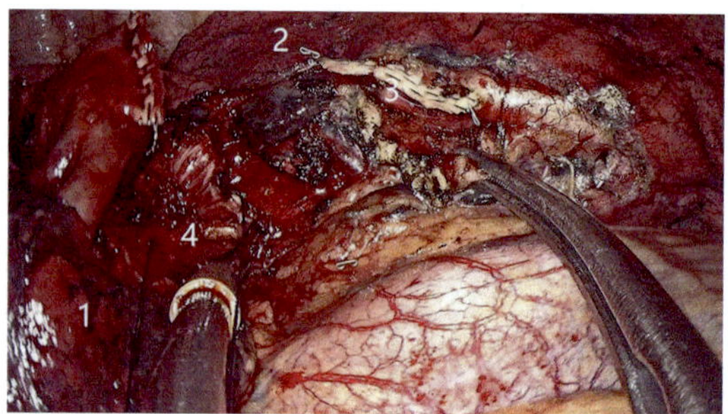

Fig. 5.18 1—Upper lobe of left lung, 2—lower lobe of left lung, 3—lower lobe artery stump of left lung, 4—bronchial stump of left lower lobe of left lung. Suture the left inferior lobar bronchial stump continuously

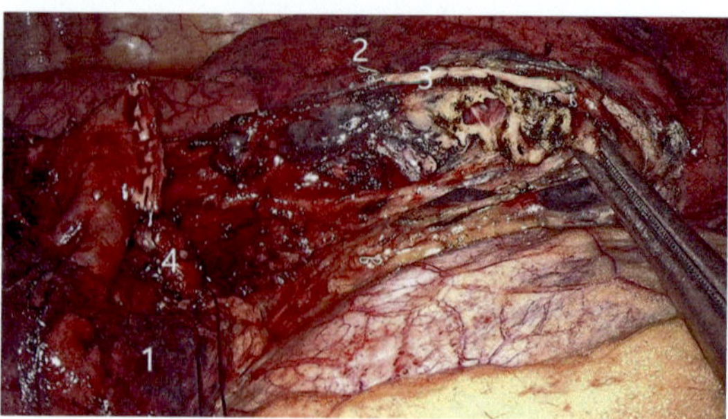

Fig. 5.19 1—Upper lobe of left lung, 2—lower lobe of left lung, 3—lower lobe artery stump of left lung, 4—bronchial stump of left lower lobe of left lung. Finished stitching

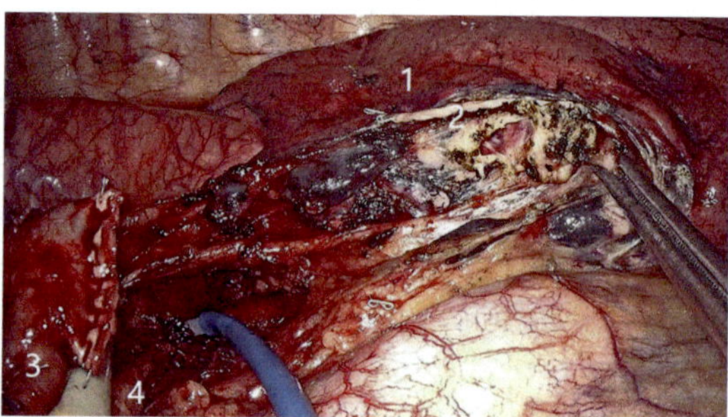

Fig. 5.20 1—Lower lobe of the left lung, 2—stump of the lower lobe artery of the left lung, 3—artery of the upper lobe of the left lung, 4—left main bronchus. It follows the left main bronchus down to the anterior esophagus

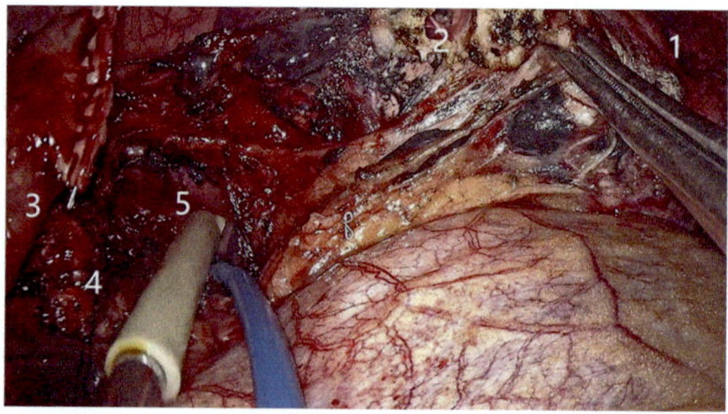

Fig. 5.21 1—Lower lobe of left lung, 2—bronchial stump of lower lobe of left lung, 3—lingual artery of upper lobe of left lung, 4—main bronchus of left lung, 5—esophagus. Sweep down the anterior esophagus

The dissection of the left subprotuberant lymph nodes is a difficult point in radical resection of lung cancer. In this case, the whole lymph node was removed from the top down, and the lower pulmonary vein was severed at the end to maintain the downward pulling of the lung tissue during the whole process, which was conducive to the exposure of the subprotuberant lymph nodes.

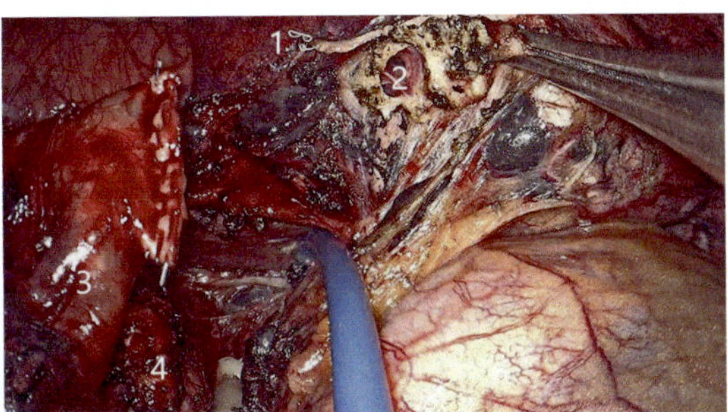

Fig. 5.22 1—Lower lobe of the left lung, 2—stump of the bronchus of the lower lobe of the left lung, 3—artery of the lingual segment of the upper lobe of the left lung, 4—left main bronchus. Sweep down the right side of the esophagus

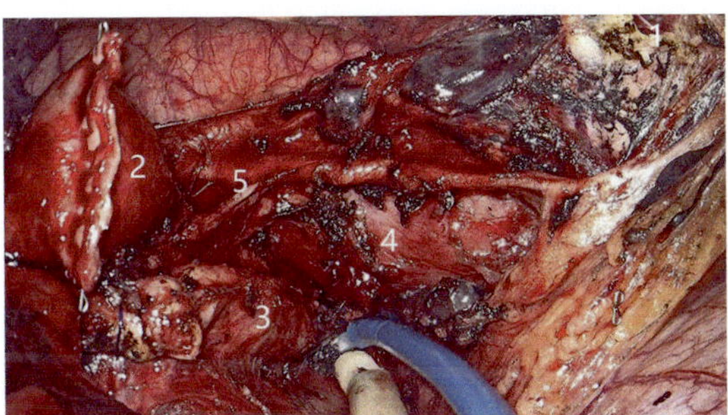

Fig. 5.23 1—Lower lobe of left lung, 2—main bronchus interlobar trunk of left pulmonary artery, 3—left main bronchus, 4—esophagus, 5—vagus nerve. Sweep down the left main bronchus

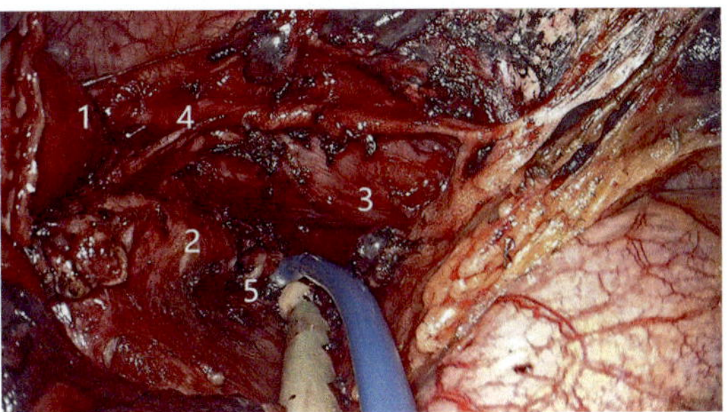

Fig. 5.24 1—Left pulmonary interlobar trunk, 2—left main bronchus, 3—esophagus, 4—vagus nerve, 5—right main bronchus. The right main bronchus was exposed

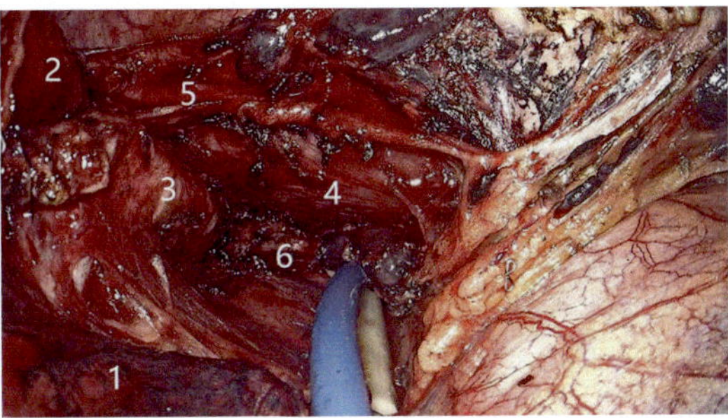

Fig. 5.25 1—Upper lobe of left lung, 2—trunk interlobar of left pulmonary artery, 3—left main bronchus, 4—esophagus, 5—vagus nerve, 6—right main bronchus. Sweep down the right main bronchus

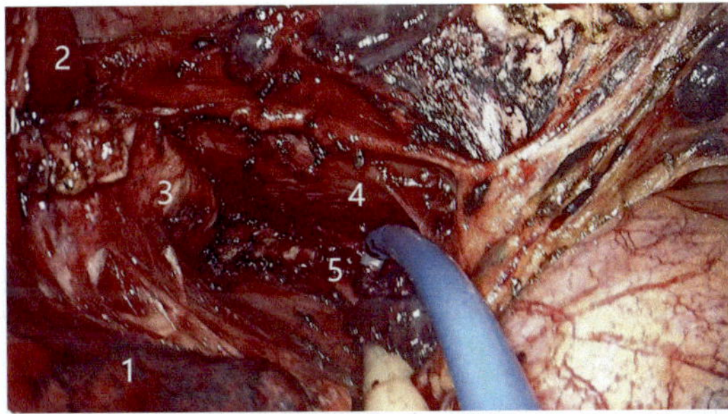

Fig. 5.26 1—Upper lobe of left lung, 2—trunk interlobar of left pulmonary artery, 3—left main bronchus, 4—esophagus, 5—right main bronchus. The right middle segment bronchial lymph nodes were cleared and the lymph nodes in the subcarina region were cleared

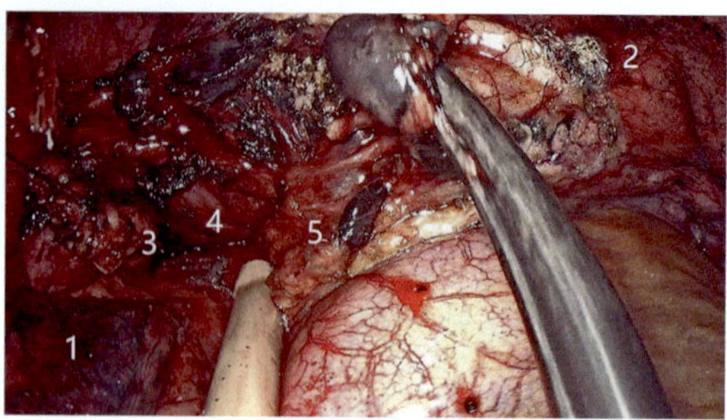

Fig. 5.27 1—Upper lobe of left lung, 2—lower lobe of left lung, 3—main bronchus, 4—esophagus, 5—vein of lower lobe of left lung. Lymph nodes above and behind the left inferior lobe were dissected

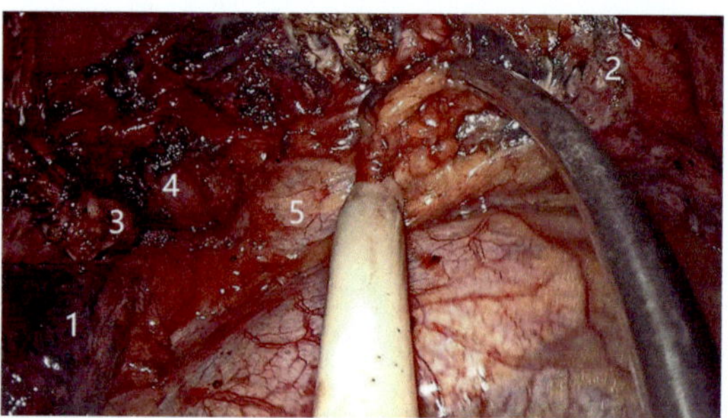

Fig. 5.28 1—Upper lobe of left lung, 2—lower lobe of left lung, 3—main bronchus, 4—esophagus, 5—vein of lower lobe of left lung. Lymph nodes in anterior inferior lobe of left lung were dissected

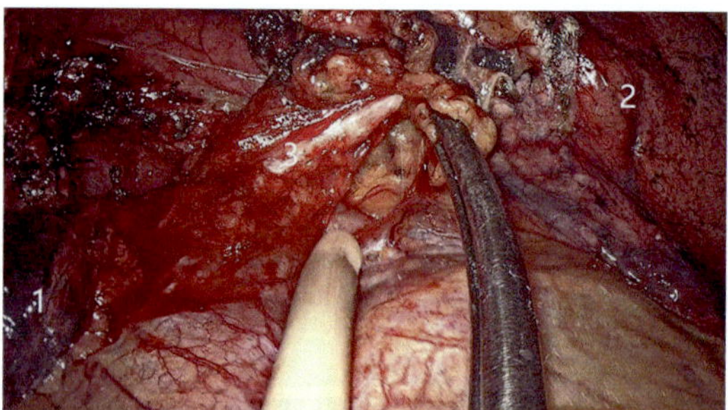

Fig. 5.29 1—Upper lobe of left lung, 2—lower lobe of left lung, 3—lower lobe vein of left lung. Free left inferior pulmonary vein

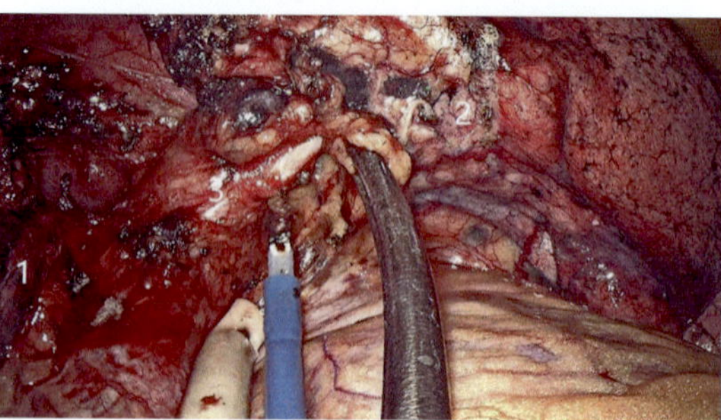

Fig. 5.30 1—Upper lobe of left lung, 2—lower lobe of left lung, 3—vein of lower lobe of left lung. Lymph nodes below and behind the left inferior lobe vein were cleared

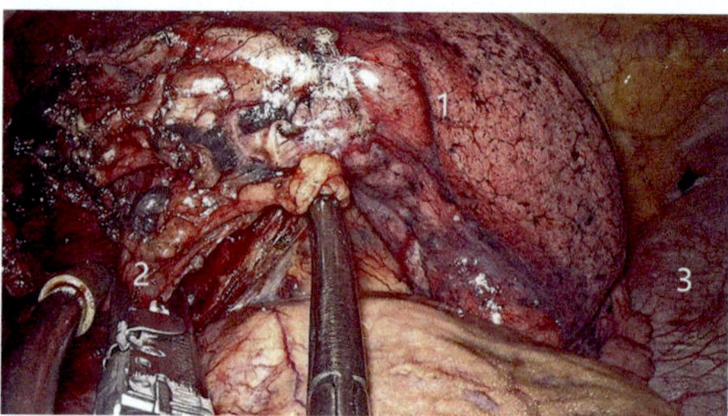

Fig. 5.31 1—Lower lobe of left lung, 2—lower lobe vein of left lung, 3—diaphragmatic muscle. GIA was used to dissect the left inferior lobe vein at the root

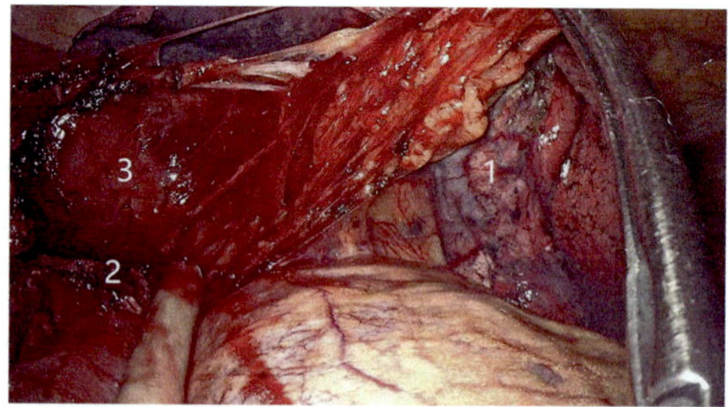

Fig. 5.32 1—Left inferior lobe, 2—left inferior lobe venous stump, 3—esophagus. Sweep down the anterior esophagus below the left inferior pulmonary vein

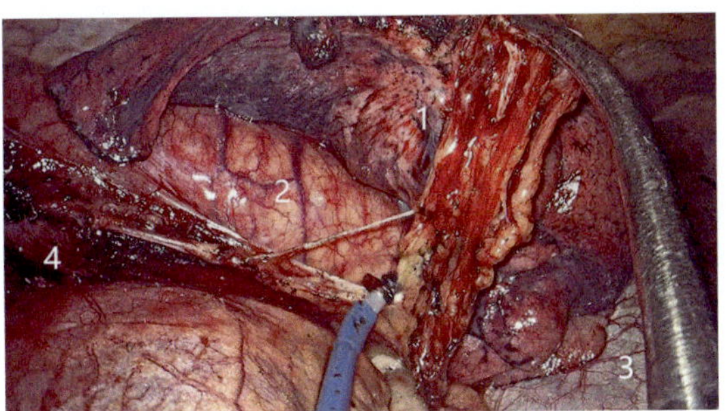

Fig. 5.33 1—Lower lobe of left lung, 2—descending aorta, 3—diaphragm, 4—esophagus. Lymph nodes in the lower lung ligament area were removed

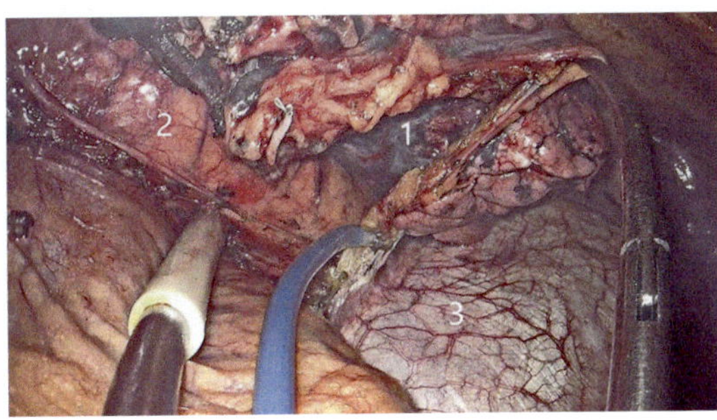

Fig. 5.34 1—Lower lobe of left lung, 2—descending aorta, 3—diaphragm. Severed the lower lung ligaments and completed the lobectomy

Surgical features Summary: Resection of the left inferior lobe of the lung is relatively simple in thoracoscopic lobectomy. In this case, the method of total resection of regional lymph nodes was also adopted. During the operation, after the suture of the left inferior lobar bronchus was completed, the suture was pulled, which played a good role in exposing the left main bronchus and the carina area. Lymph node dissection in the pulmonary fenestrum area can be seen in the chapter on the upper lobe of the left lung, which is not discussed in this chapter.

Part II

Exaltation Chapter

The difficulty in thoracoscopic lobectomy often lies in the separation difficulty caused by the lymph nodes surrounding the blood vessels and bronchus. There are different ways to solve this problem. In the improvement part, we show one method to solve this difficulty: The case of right inferior lobe resection in this study was a patient after TKI adjuvant therapy, with multiple hyperplasia and enlargement of lymph nodes, dense adhesion to the surrounding tissue, and difficult separation. Normal anatomical space can be found by the method of anatomical separation from normal tissue to tumor tissue, and the lymph and tumor tissues can be completely removed, avoiding the accident caused by direct separation of tumors along the outer edge of the tumor and blind separation. Complete resection of tumor has always been one of the first principles of tumor surgery. This article perfectly explains how to achieve this principle. I believe readers will benefit a lot from it.

6 Excision of the Right Inferior Lobe of Lung

Electric hook is widely used in thoracoscopic surgery. It is relatively long, but its distal stability is also poor because of its length. Compared with electrotome, it has its advantages and disadvantages, and the use of it depends entirely on the preferences of the surgeon.

This is cases of progression after TKI treatment.

A middle-aged male patient was admitted to the hospital with a dry cough for 1 month; admission CT.

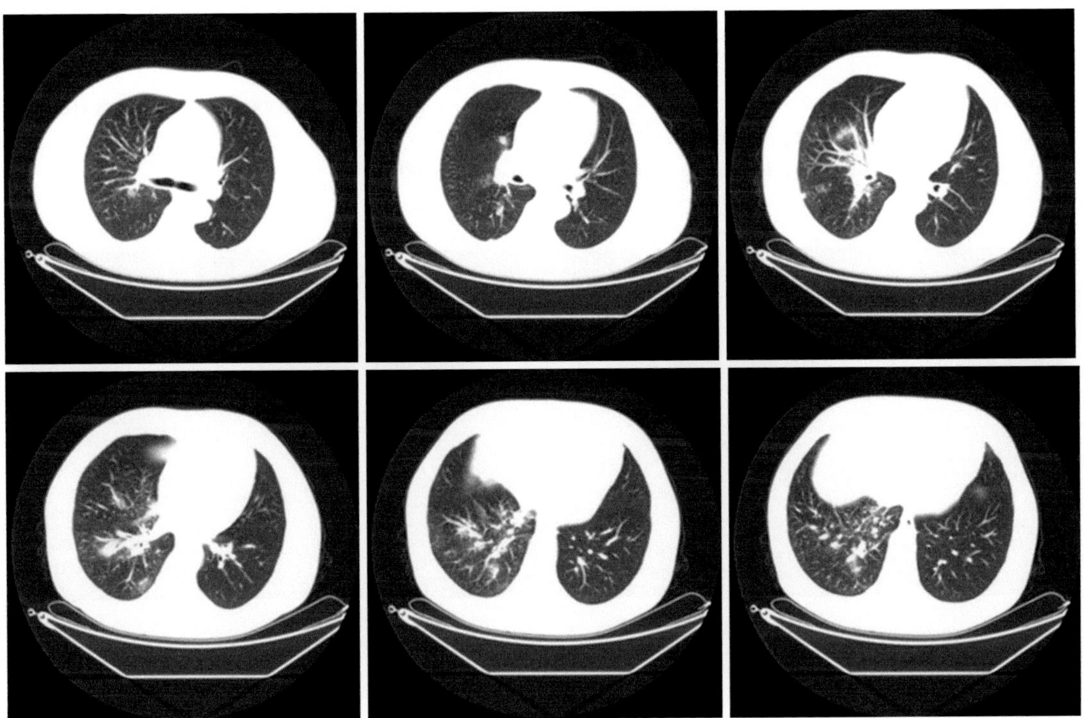

J. Li, Z. Long, *Atlas of Thoracoscopic Lobectomy with Bronchoplasty*,
https://doi.org/10.1007/978-981-99-5150-5_6

EBUS-TBNA biopsy was performed after admission and pathological findings showed adenocarcinoma of the lung with genetic testing.

CHART-test results and medication tips

Variant gene	Form of mutation/ frequency of mutation	FDA/CFDA certified				Other clinical study-stage drugs
		Similar cancers	Sensitivity projections	Other cancers	Sensitivity projections	
EGFR	p._745 750del (27.65%) accompanied gene amplification	Gefitinib	Sensitive			Dacomitinib
		Erlotinib	Sensitive			XL647
		Icotinib	Sensitive			AZD3759
		Afatinib	Sensitive			
		Osimertinib (AZD9291)	Sensitive			
TP53	p.R175H (7.31%)					MPK-0917-AAG
						Ganetespib
						AZD1775
						APR-246
						ALT-801
						SGT-53
						Alisertib
						AT9283
						ENMD-2076
						AMG 900

- The patient was treated with Icotinib 125 mg/tid and reviewed every 2 months, review after 6 months showed tumor progression, and right inferior lobectomy was performed (Figs. 6.1, 6.2, 6.3, 6.4, 6.5, 6.6, 6.7, 6.8, 6.9, and 6.10).

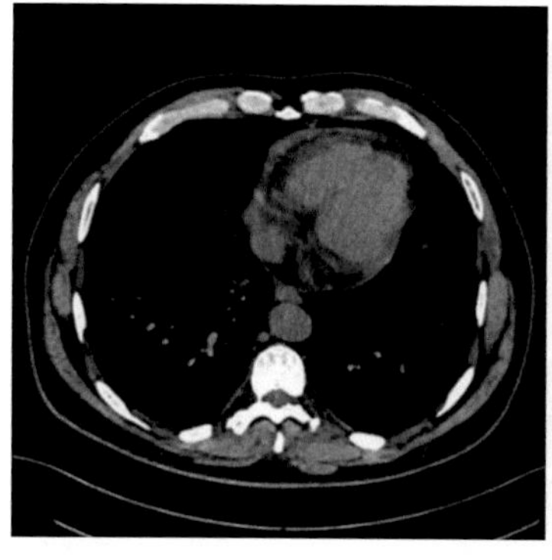

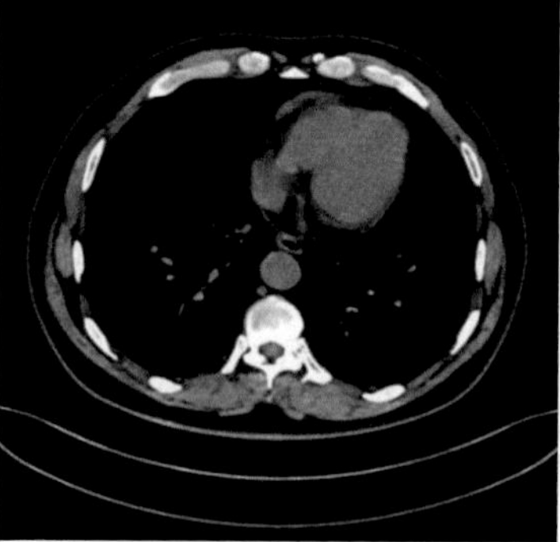

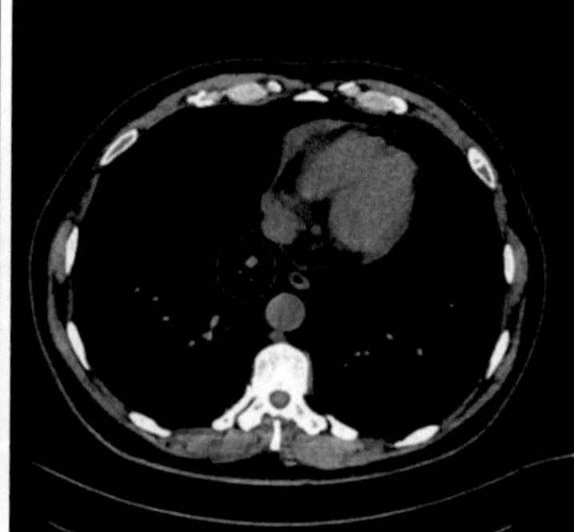

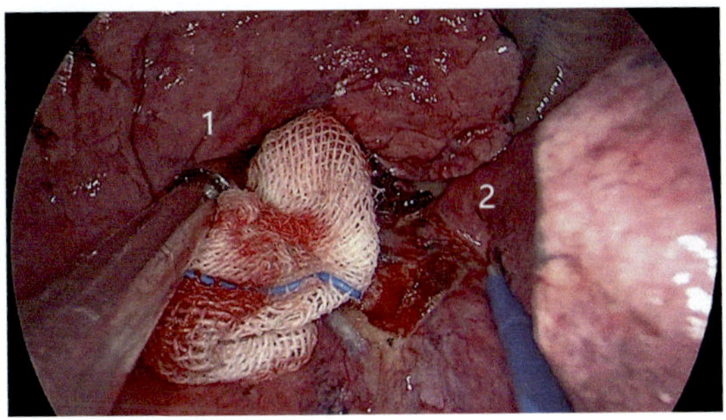

Fig. 6.1 1—Inferior lobe of right lung, 2—superior lobe of right lung. Open interlobar fissure

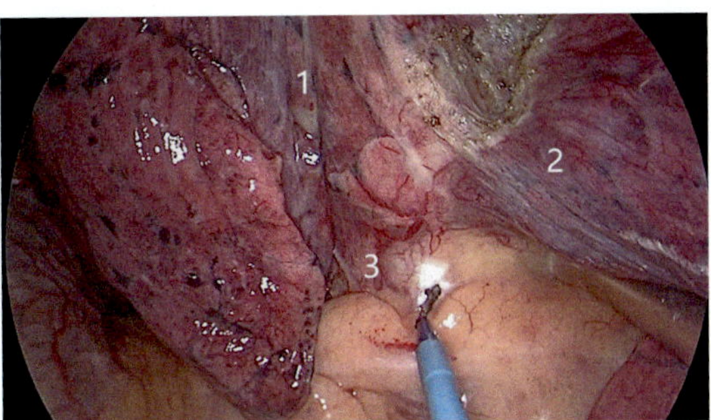

Fig. 6.4 1—Inferior lobe of right lung, 2—middle lobe of right lung, 3—right inferior pulmonary vein. Dissect along the anterior right inferior pulmonary vein

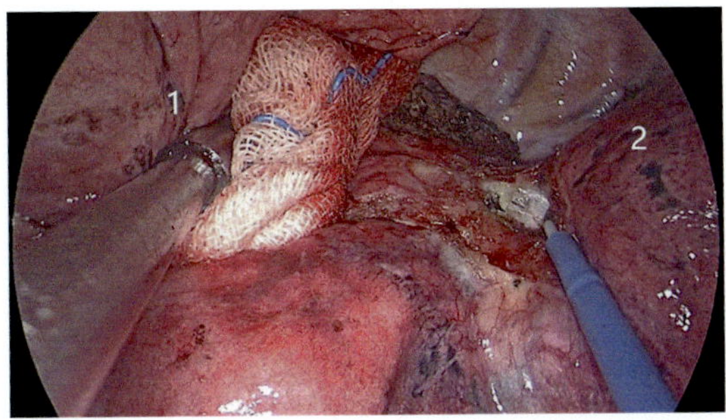

Fig. 6.2 1—Inferior lobe of right lung, 2—superior lobe of right lung. The interlobar fissure was frozen like, near to superior lobe of right lung, dissect interlobular fissures and reveal interlobular vessels

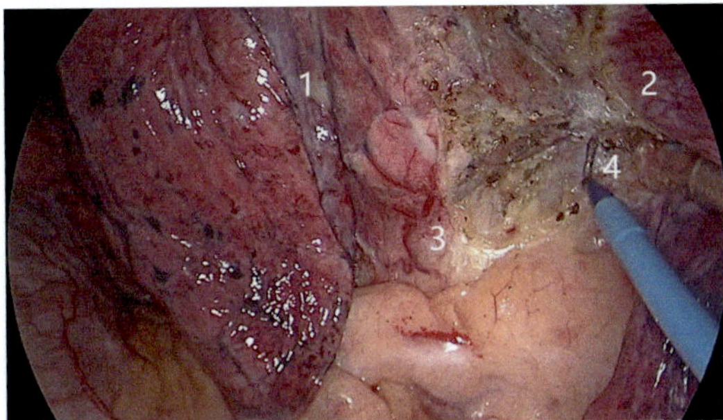

Fig. 6.5 1—Inferior lobe of right lung, 2—middle lobe of right lung, 3—right inferior pulmonary vein, 4—right middle pulmonary vein. Reveal right middle pulmonary vein and dissect the interlobar fissure along the surface of right middle pulmonary vein

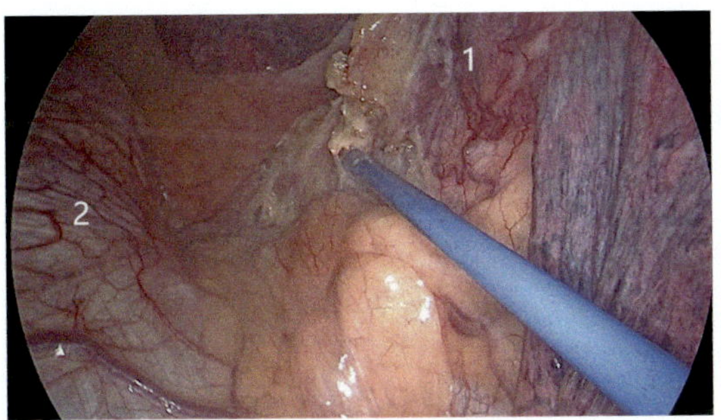

Fig. 6.3 1—Inferior lobe of right lung, 2—diaphragm. Cut off inferior pulmonary ligament

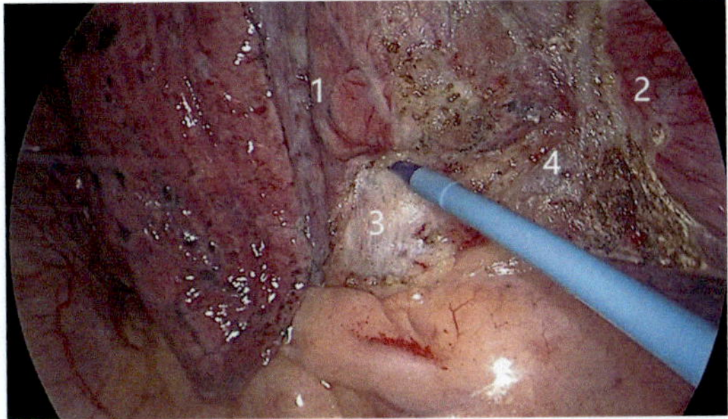

Fig. 6.6 1—Inferior lobe of right lung, 2—superior lobe of right lung, 3—right inferior pulmonary vein, 4—right middle pulmonary vein. Dissect the anterior right inferior pulmonary vein

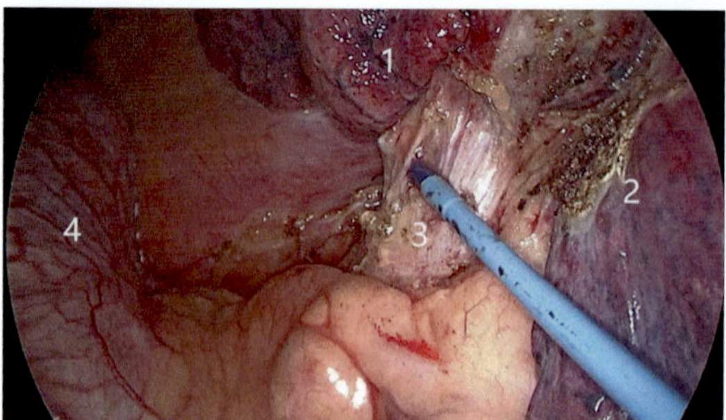

Fig. 6.7 1—Inferior lobe of right lung, 2—middle lobe of right lung, 3—right inferior pulmonary vein, 4—diaphragm. Dissect the posterior and inferior right inferior pulmonary vein

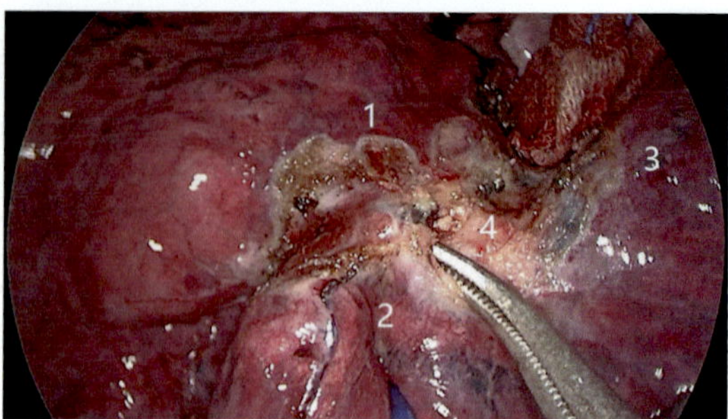

Fig. 6.10 1—Inferior lobe of right lung, 2—middle lobe of right lung, 3—superior lobe of right lung, 4—interlobar trunk of right pulmonary artery. Dissect along the inferior middle lobe of right lung at the intersection of interlobar fissure

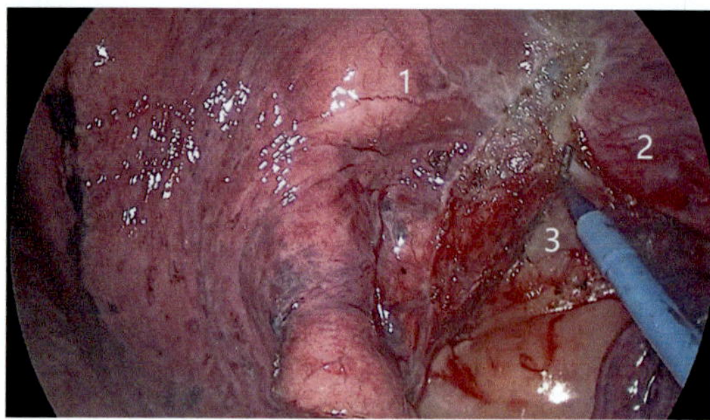

Fig. 6.8 1—Inferior lobe of right lung, 2—middle lobe of right lung, 3—right middle pulmonary vein. Open interlobar fissure below the middle lobe of right lung, in front of right middle pulmonary vein

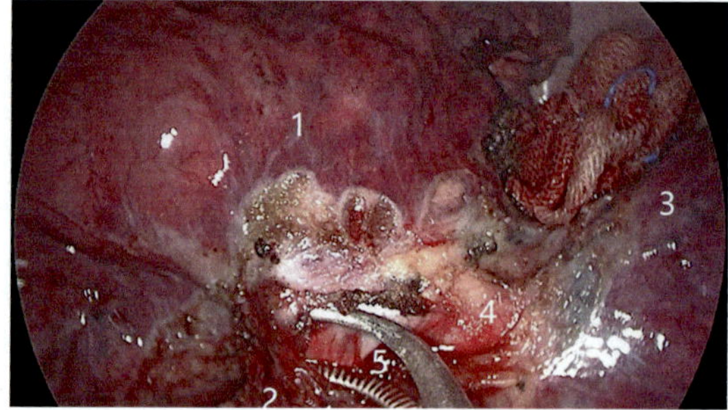

Fig. 6.11 1—Inferior lobe of right lung, 2—middle lobe of right lung, 3—superior lobe of right lung, 4—interlobar trunk of right pulmonary artery, 5—right middle pulmonary artery. Reveal right middle lobe lateral segment artery and open interlobar fissure in front of it

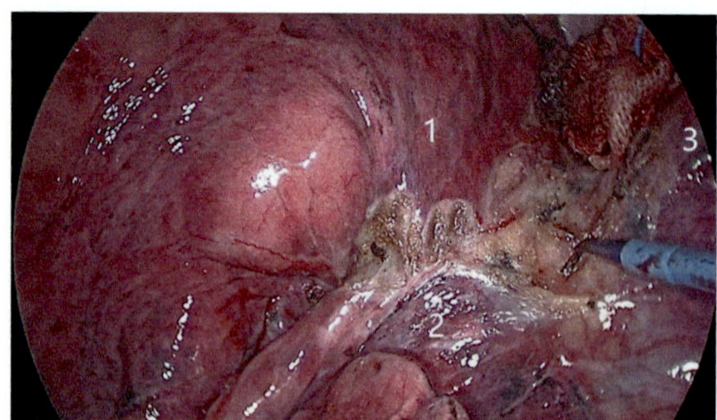

Fig. 6.9 1—Inferior lobe of right lung, 2—middle lobe of right lung, 3—superior lobe of right lung. Dissect the interlobar fissure backward to forward until the intersection of inferior lobe of right lung and middle lobe of right lung

Surgical features: In this case, the disease progressed after 6 months of TKI treatment. During the operation, the pulmonary hilar adhesion was severe and the structure was unclear. The separation started from the relatively normal part of the structure, revealing important anatomical structures such as the pulmonary trunk and bronchus, and then from the far to the near, revealing the inferior pulmonary artery branches and bronchus (Figs. 6.11, 6.12, 6.13, 6.14, 6.15, 6.16, 6.17, 6.18, 6.19, 6.20, 6.21, 6.22, 6.23, 6.24, 6.25, 6.26, 6.27, 6.28, 6.29, 6.30, 6.31, 6.32, 6.33, 6.34, 6.35, 6.36, 6.37, 6.38, 6.39, 6.40, 6.41, 6.42, 6.43, 6.44, 6.45, 6.46, 6.47, 6.48, 6.49, 6.50, 6.51, 6.52, 6.53, and 6.54).

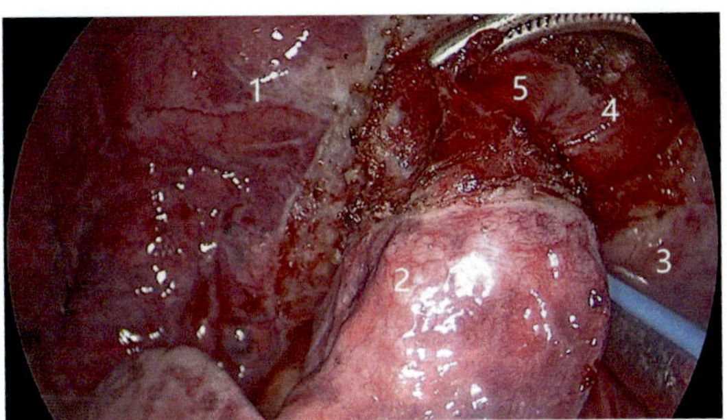

Fig. 6.12 1—Superior lobe of right lung, 2—middle lobe of right lung, 3—superior lobe of right lung, 4—interlobar trunk of right pulmonary artery, 5—right middle lobe lateral segment artery. Dissect right middle lobe lateral segment artery

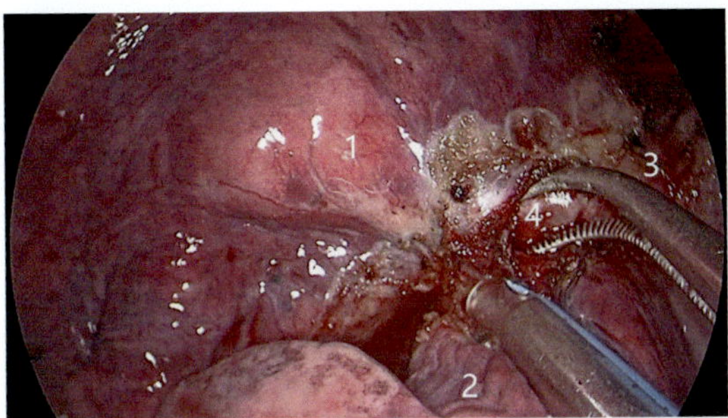

Fig. 6.13 1—Inferior lobe of right lung, 2—middle lobe of right lung, 3—superior lobe of right lung, 4—right inferior lobe basal segment artery. Dissect along right middle lobe lateral segment artery downward and reveal right inferior lobe basal segment artery

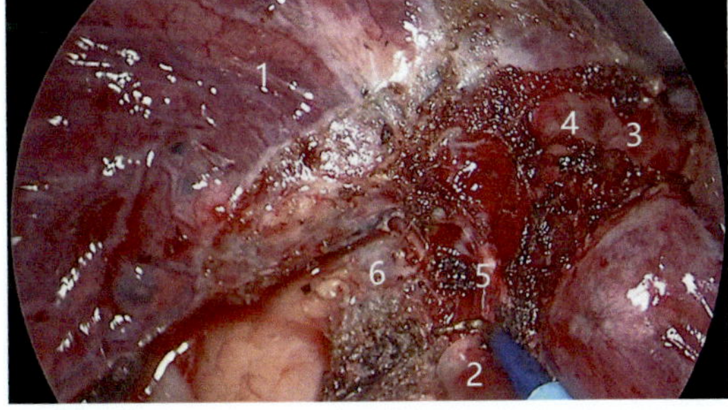

Fig. 6.14 1—Inferior lobe of right lung, 2—middle lobe of right lung, 3—superior lobe of right lung, 4—right middle lobe lateral segment artery, 5—right middle lobar bronchus, 6—right inferior pulmonary vein. Dissect anterior right middle lobe lateral segment artery and reveal right middle lobar bronchus

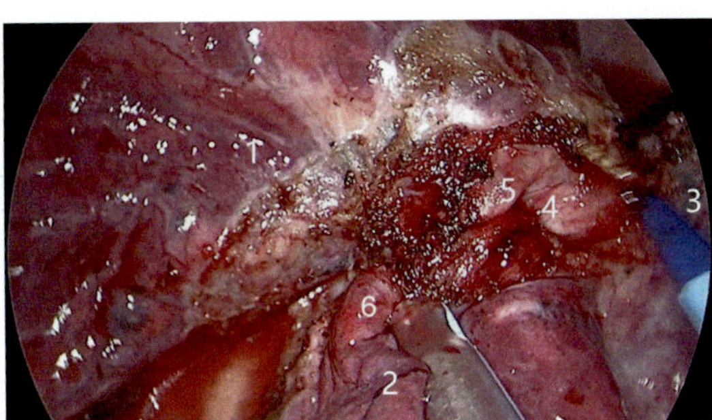

Fig. 6.15 1—Inferior lobe of right lung, 2—middle lobe of right lung, 3—superior lobe of right lung, 4—right middle lobe lateral segment artery, 5—right middle lobar bronchus, 6—right inferior pulmonary vein. Dissect anterior right middle lobe lateral segment artery and reveal right middle lobar bronchus

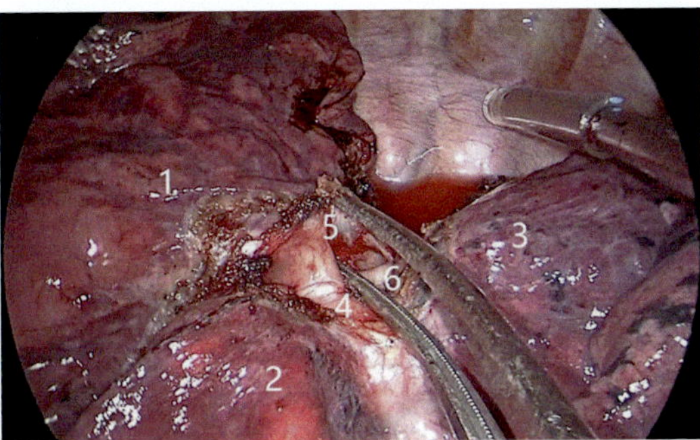

Fig. 6.16 1—Inferior lobe of right lung, 2—middle lobe of right lung, 3—superior lobe of right lung, 4—interlobar trunk of right pulmonary artery, 5—dorsal segment artery of inferior lobe of right lung, 6—posterior segment artery of superior lobe of right lung. Reveal the beginning of dorsal segment artery of inferior lobe of right lung

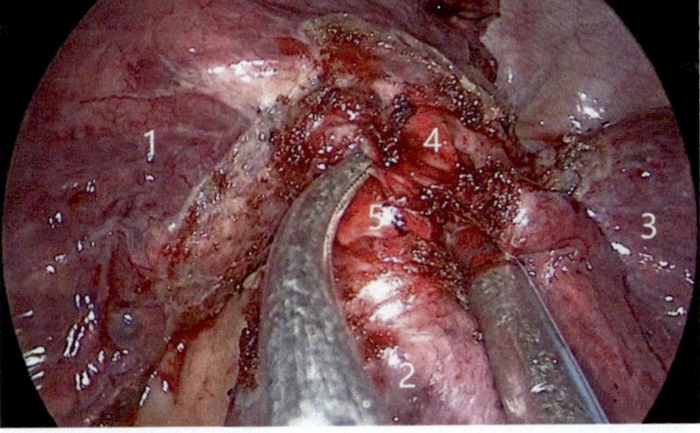

Fig. 6.17 1—Inferior lobe of right lung, 2—middle lobe of right lung, 3—superior lobe of right lung right middle lobe lateral segment artery, 4—right middle lobe lateral segment artery, 5—right middle lobar bronchus. Dissect the lymph node along right middle lobar bronchus downward

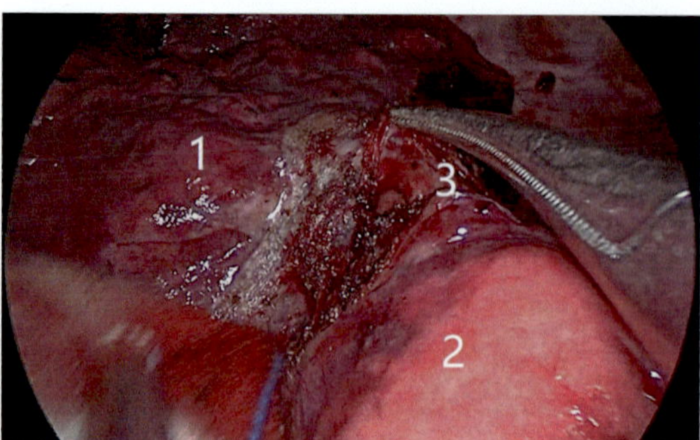

Fig. 6.18 1—Inferior lobe of right lung, 2—middle lobe of right lung, 3—right middle lobe lateral segment artery. Dissect right middle lobe lateral segment artery downward

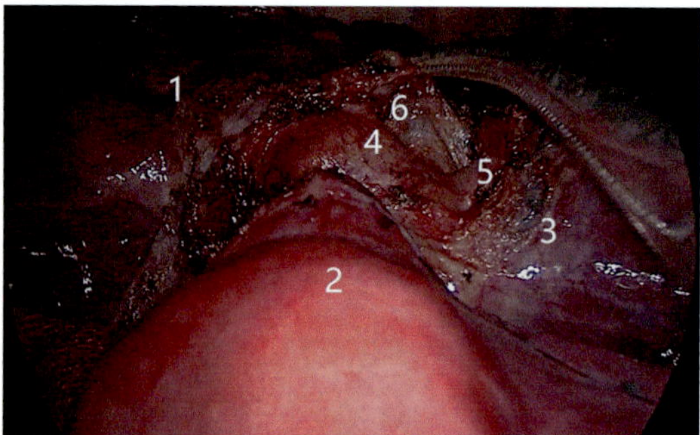

Fig. 6.19 1—Inferior lobe of right lung, 2—middle lobe of right lung, 3—superior lobe of right lung, 4—interlobar trunk of right pulmonary artery, 5—posterior segment artery of superior lobe of right lung, 6—dorsal segment artery of inferior lobe of right lung. Dissect the dorsal segment artery of inferior lobe of right lung and reveal the lymphoid tissue behind it

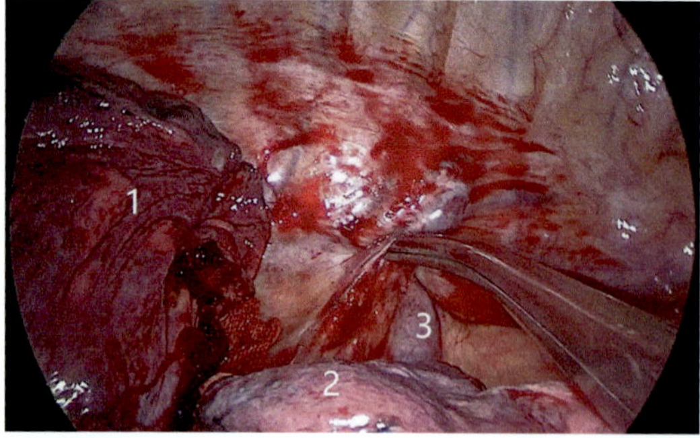

Fig. 6.20 1—Inferior lobe of right lung, 2—middle lobe of right lung, 3—arch of azygos vein. Open the mediastinum pleura along the inferior arch of azygos vein

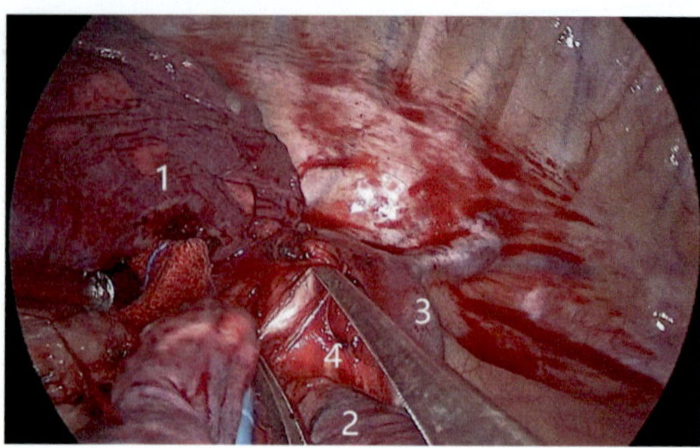

Fig. 6.21 1—Inferior lobe of right lung, 2—middle lobe of right lung, 3—arch of azygos vein, 4—right superior lobar bronchus. Dissect along right superior lobar bronchus backward and downward

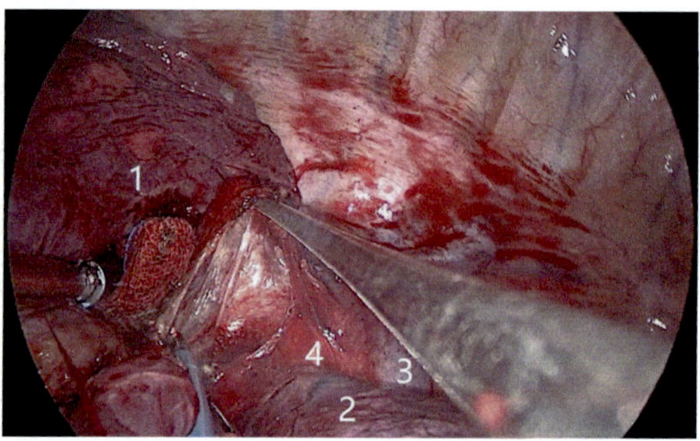

Fig. 6.22 1—Inferior lobe of right lung, 2—middle lobe of right lung, 3—arch of azygos vein, 4—right superior lobar bronchus. Reveal the lymphoid tissue behind and below the right superior lobar bronchus

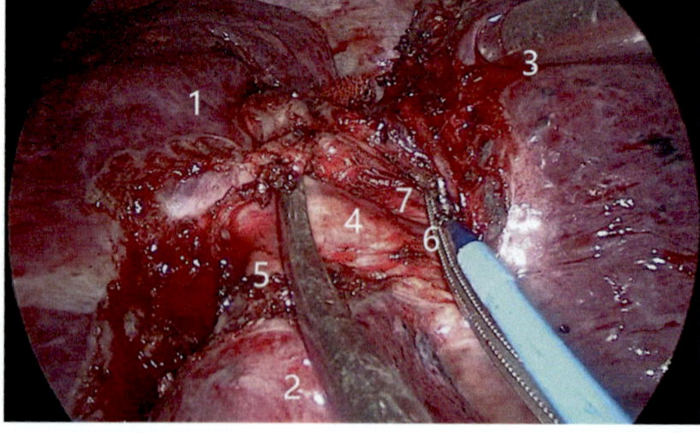

Fig. 6.23 1—Inferior lobe of right lung, 2—middle lobe of right lung, 3—superior lobe of right lung, 4—interlobar trunk of right pulmonary artery, 5—right middle lobe lateral segment artery, 6—posterior segment artery of superior lobe of right lung, 7—right middle segment bronchus. Dissect the posterior interlobar trunk of right pulmonary artery and connect to the lymphoid tissues dissected behind and below the right superior lobar bronchus

Summary: This case demonstrates a salvage procedure for progression after TKI treatment, which is significantly more difficult and difficult to separate between the normal anatomic gaps. The atlas cannot fully demonstrate the delicacy and skill of this procedure, and the reader can refer to the surgical video to appreciate the subtlety of the procedure.

The characteristics of this case are that the dissection starts from the margins of the right upper lobe and right middle lobe of the lung, which emphasizes the radical surgery and allows dissection in a relatively lightly adherent area, which is safer; the lymph node dissection of the upper mediastinum can be found in the Chap. 2 "Upper Lobe of the Right Lung" and Chap. 3 "Middle Lobe of the Right Lung," which will not be repeated in this chapter.

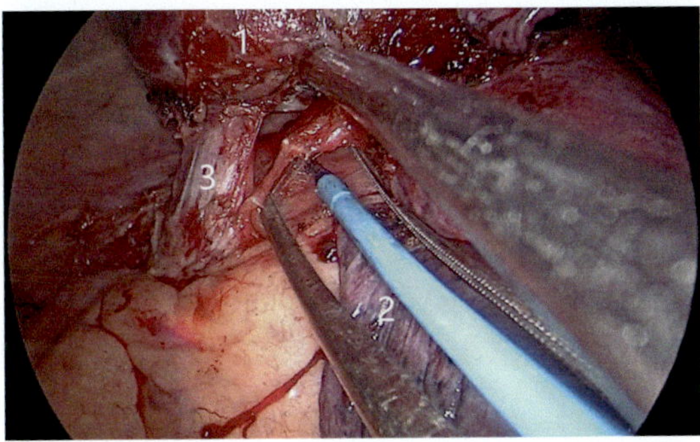

Fig. 6.24 1—Inferior lobe of right lung, 2—middle lobe of right lung, 3—right inferior pulmonary vein. Dissect right inferior pulmonary vein and lymphoid tissues above it

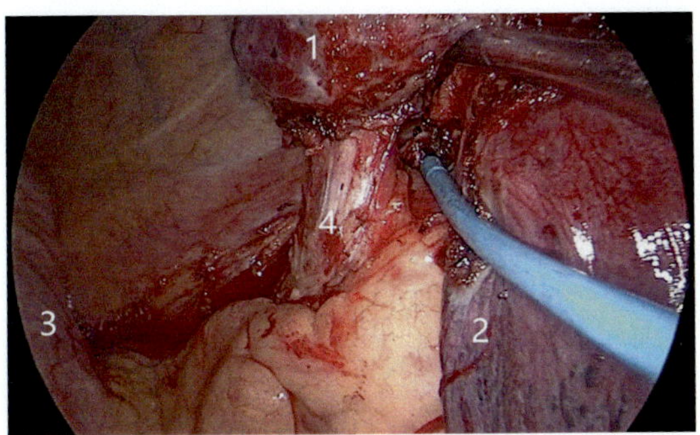

Fig. 6.25 1—Inferior lobe of right lung, 2—middle lobe of right lung, 3—diaphragm, 4—right inferior pulmonary vein. Continue to dissect along superior right inferior pulmonary vein upward and connect to the lymphoid tissues dissected, finish the dissection behind the hilum

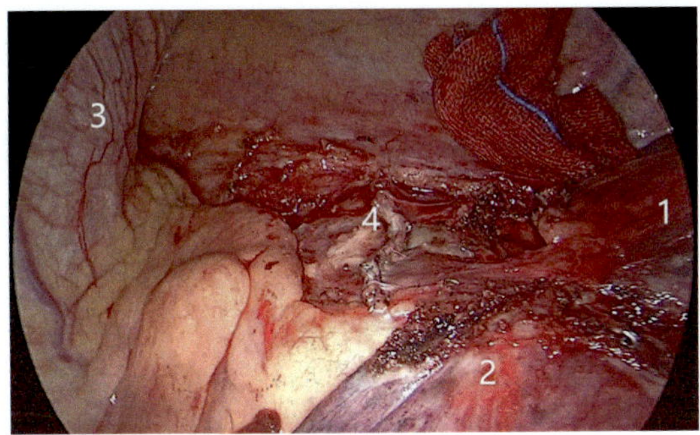

Fig. 6.26 1—Inferior lobe of right lung, 2—middle lobe of right lung, 3—diaphragm, 4—right inferior pulmonary vein stump. Interrupt right inferior pulmonary vein with GIA

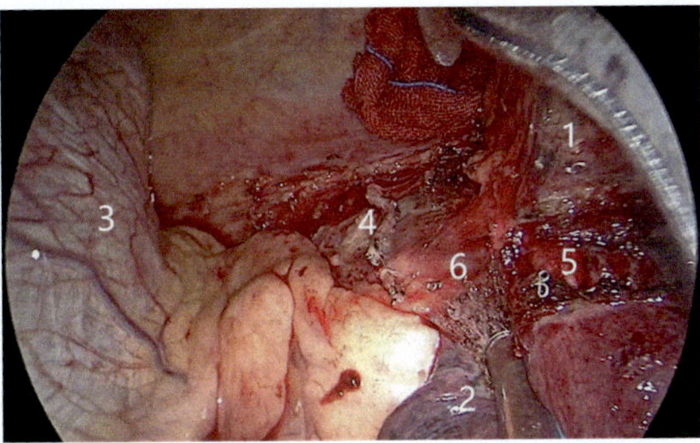

Fig. 6.27 1—Inferior lobe of right lung, 2—middle lobe of right lung, 3—diaphragm, 4—right inferior pulmonary vein stump, 5—right middle lobe lateral segment artery, 6—right middle pulmonary vein. Reveal the right middle pulmonary vein

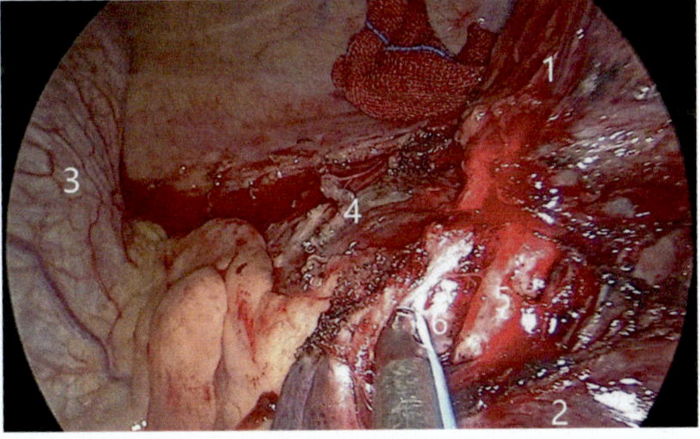

Fig. 6.28 1—Inferior lobe of right lung, 2—middle lobe of right lung, 3—diaphragm, 4—right inferior pulmonary vein stump, 5—right middle lobe lateral segment artery, 6—right middle pulmonary vein. Open adventitia of right middle pulmonary vein and dissect right middle lobar bronchus backward and upward to reveal

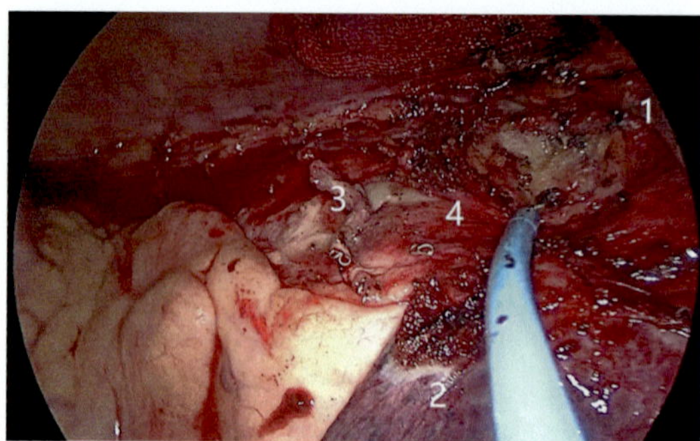

Fig. 6.29 1—Inferior lobe of right lung, 2—middle lobe of right lung, 3—right inferior pulmonary vein stump, 4—pericardium. Dissect along pericardium backward and upward

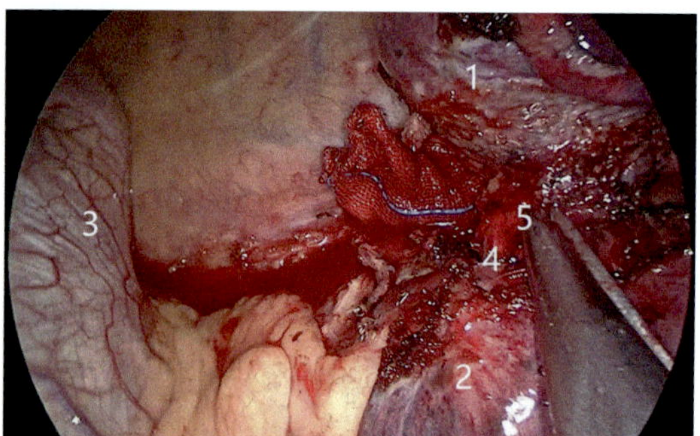

Fig. 6.30 1—Inferior lobe of right lung, 2—middle lobe of right lung, 3—diaphragm, 4—right middle lobar bronchus, 5—right inferior lobar bronchus. Dissect along right middle lobar bronchus backward and reveal right inferior lobar bronchus

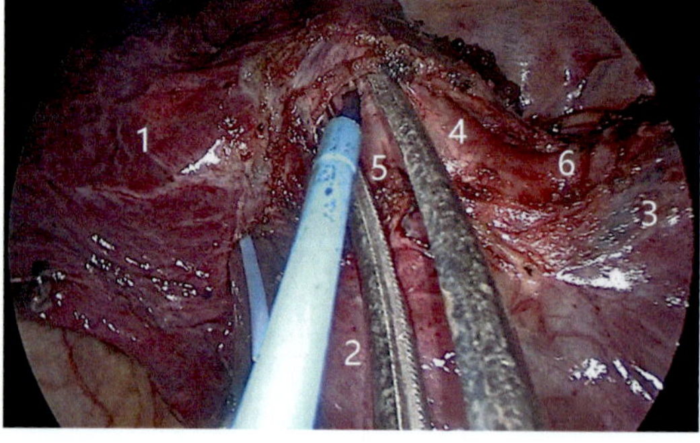

Fig. 6.31 1—Inferior lobe of right lung, 2—middle lobe of right lung, 3—superior lobe of right lung, 4—interlobar trunk of right pulmonary artery, 5—right middle lobe lateral segment artery, 6—dorsal segment artery of superior lobe of right lung. Dissect right inferior pulmonary artery downward along interlobar trunk of right pulmonary artery

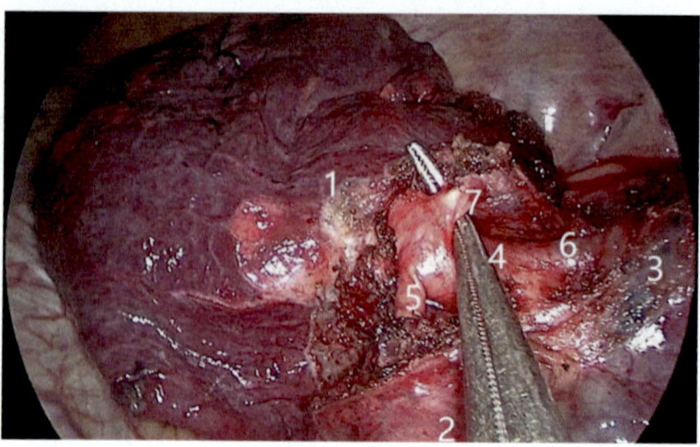

Fig. 6.32 1—Inferior lobe of right lung, 2—middle lobe of right lung, 3—superior lobe of right lung, 4—interlobar trunk of right pulmonary artery, 5—right middle lobe lateral segment artery, 6—posterior segment artery of superior lobe of right lung, 7—dorsal segment artery of inferior lobe of right lung. Dissect, ligature, and cut off dorsal segment artery of inferior lobe of right lung

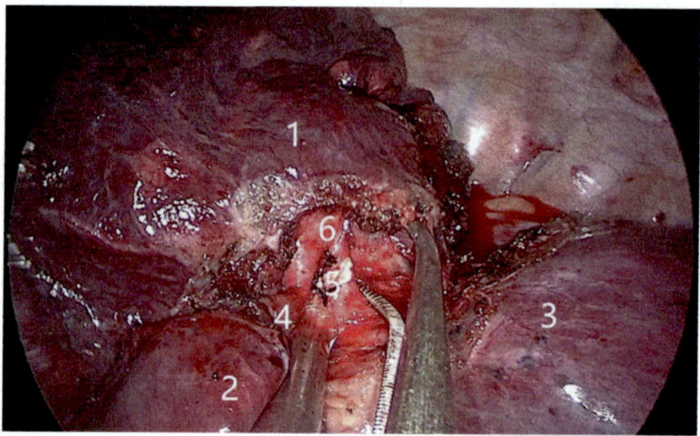

Fig. 6.33 1—Inferior lobe of right lung, 2—middle lobe of right lung, 3—superior lobe of right lung, 4—right middle lobe lateral segment artery, 5—dorsal segment artery stump of inferior lobe of right lung, 6—right inferior lobe basal segment artery

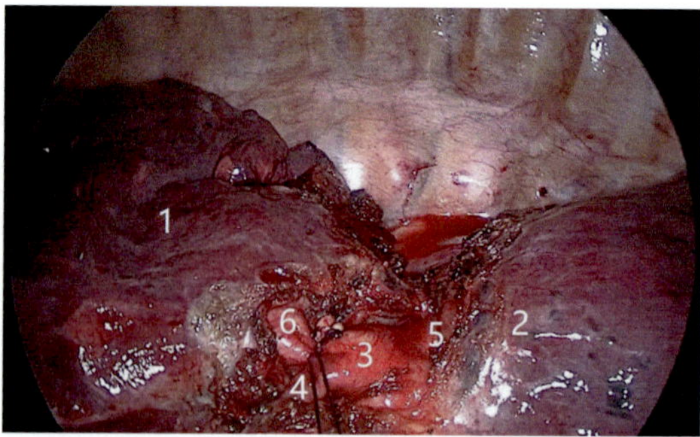

Fig. 6.34 1—Inferior lobe of right lung, 2—middle lobe of right lung, 3—interlobar trunk of right pulmonary artery, 4—right middle lobe lateral segment artery, 5—posterior segment artery of superior lobe of right lung, 6—right inferior lobe basal segment artery. Ligature right inferior lobe basal segment artery

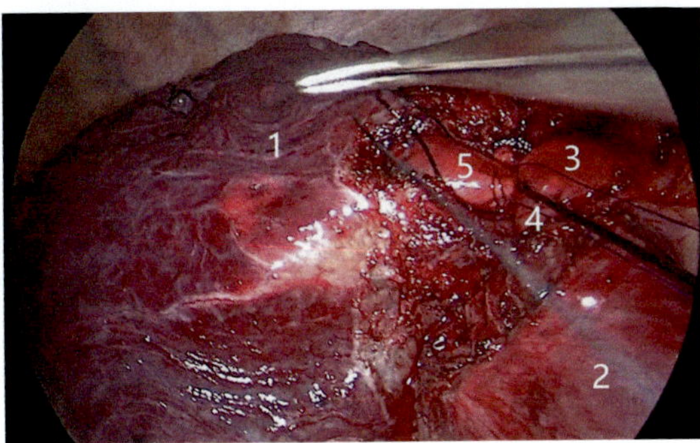

Fig. 6.35 1—Inferior lobe of right lung, 2—middle lobe of right lung, 3—interlobar trunk of right pulmonary artery, 4—right middle lobe lateral segment artery, 5—right inferior lobe basal segment artery. Suture proximal right inferior lobe basal segment artery and ligature distal end, and interrupt right inferior lobe basal segment artery

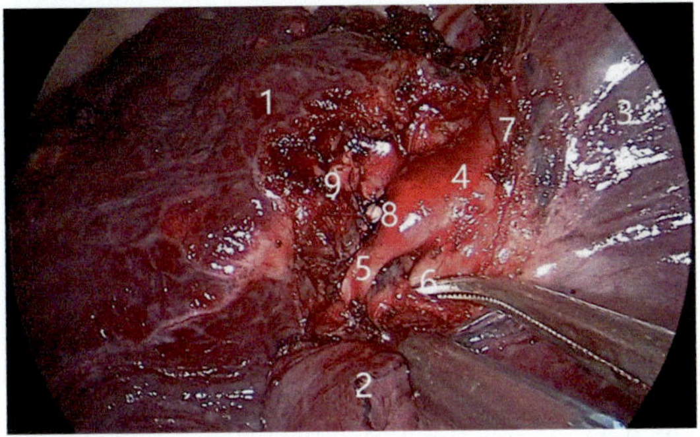

Fig. 6.36 1—Inferior lobe of right lung, 2—middle lobe of right lung, 3—superior lobe of right lung, 4—interlobar trunk of right pulmonary artery, 5—right middle lobe lateral segment artery, 6—right middle lobe medial segment artery, 7—posterior segment artery of superior lobe of right lung, 8—right inferior lobe basal segment artery proximal stump, 9—right inferior lobe basal segment artery distal stump. Dissect along interlobar trunk of right pulmonary artery forward and reveal right middle lobe medial segment artery, and dissect the lymph node behind it

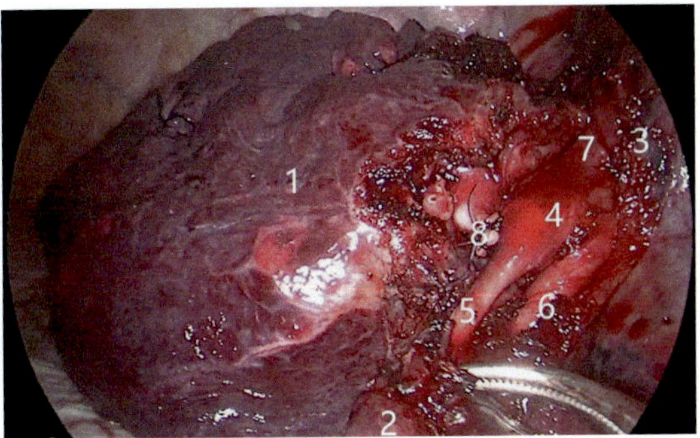

Fig. 6.37 1—Inferior lobe of right lung, 2—middle lobe of right lung, 3—superior lobe of right lung, 4—interlobar trunk of right pulmonary artery, 5—right middle lobe lateral segment artery, 6—right middle lobe medial segment artery, 7—posterior segment artery of superior lobe of right lung, 8—right inferior lobe basal segment artery proximal stump. Dissect the lymph node along right middle lobe lateral segment artery and right middle lobe medial segment artery

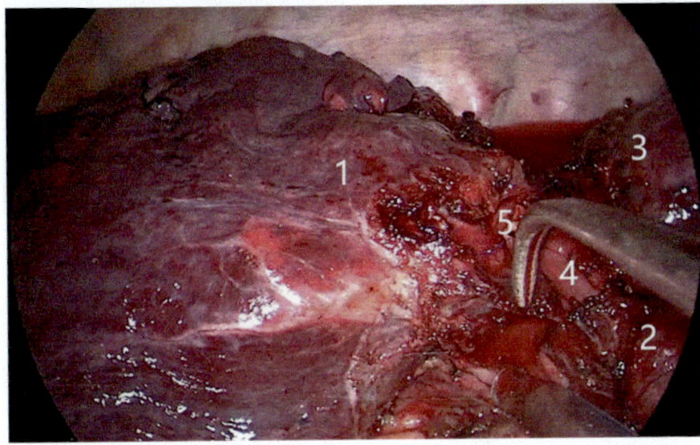

Fig. 6.38 1—Inferior lobe of right lung, 2—middle lobe of right lung, 3—superior lobe of right lung, 4—right middle lobe lateral segment artery, 5—right inferior lobe basal segment artery proximal stump. Dissect the lymph node along inferior right middle lobe lateral segment artery backward

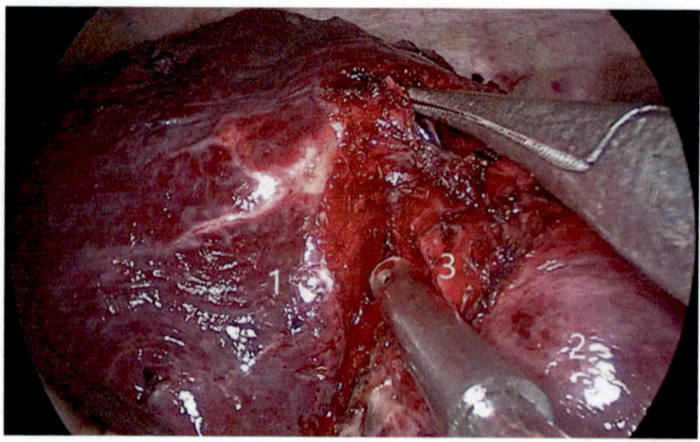

Fig. 6.39 1—Inferior lobe of right lung, 2—middle lobe of right lung, 3—right middle lobar bronchus. Dissect the lymph node along superior right middle lobar bronchus backward

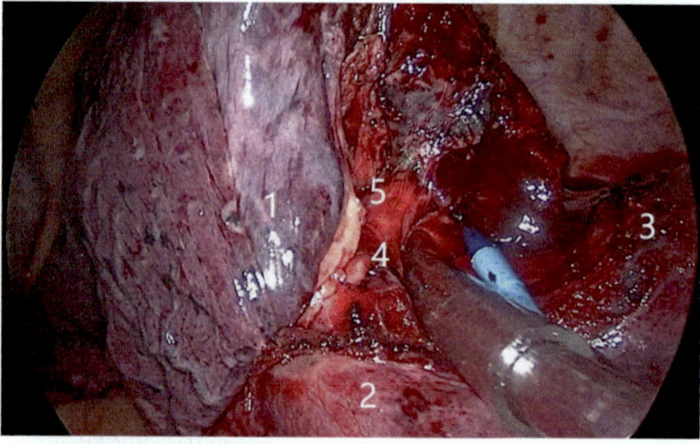

Fig. 6.40 1—Inferior lobe of right lung, 2—middle lobe of right lung, 3—superior lobe of right lung, 4—right middle lobar bronchus, 5—beginning of right inferior lobar bronchus. Dissect the lymph node along beginning of right inferior lobar bronchus

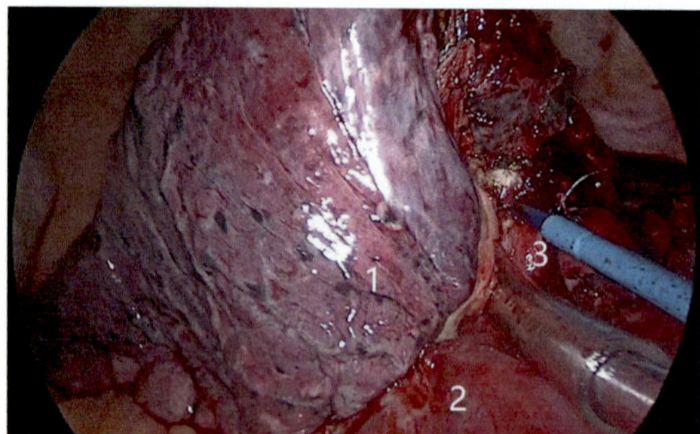

Fig. 6.41 1—Inferior lobe of right lung, 2—middle lobe of right lung, 3—right middle lobar bronchus. Cut at the opening of right inferior lobar bronchus

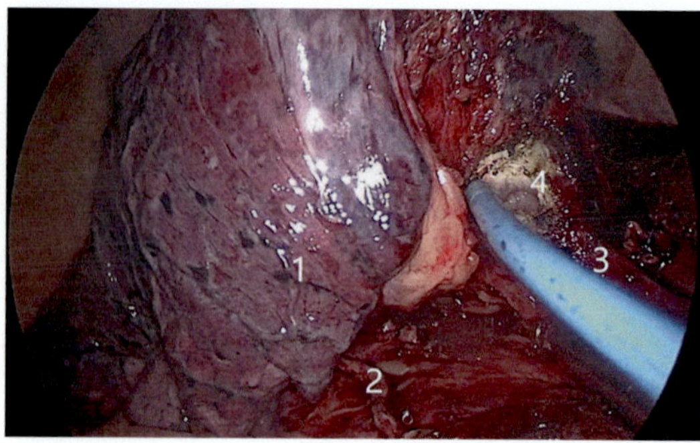

Fig. 6.42 1—Inferior lobe of right lung, 2—middle lobe of right lung, 3—right middle lobar bronchus, 4—right inferior lobar bronchial stump. Interrupt right inferior lobar bronchus at the opening of right inferior lobar bronchus

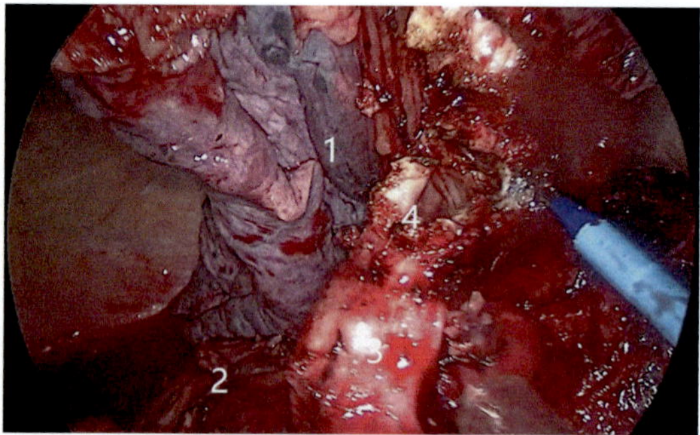

Fig. 6.43 1—Inferior lobe of right lung, 2—middle lobe of right lung, 3—right middle lobar bronchus, 4—right inferior lobar bronchial stump. Dissect the lymph node along right inferior lobar bronchial stump upward and connect to the lymph node behind the hilum

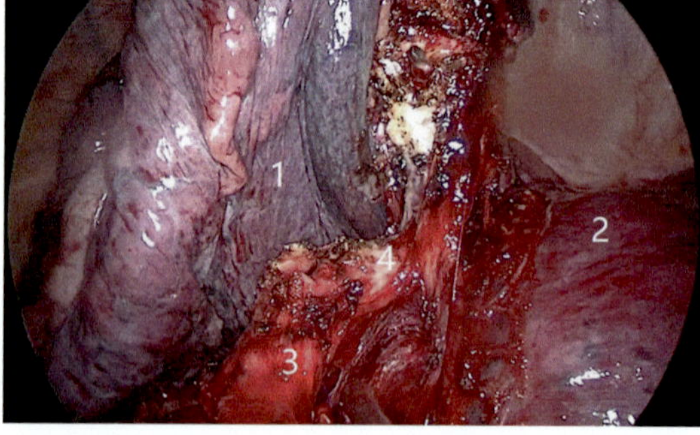

Fig. 6.44 1—Inferior lobe of right lung, 2—superior lobe of right lung, 3—right middle lobar bronchus, 4—right middle segment bronchus. Dissect the lymph node along right middle segment bronchus upward to inferior right superior lobar bronchus

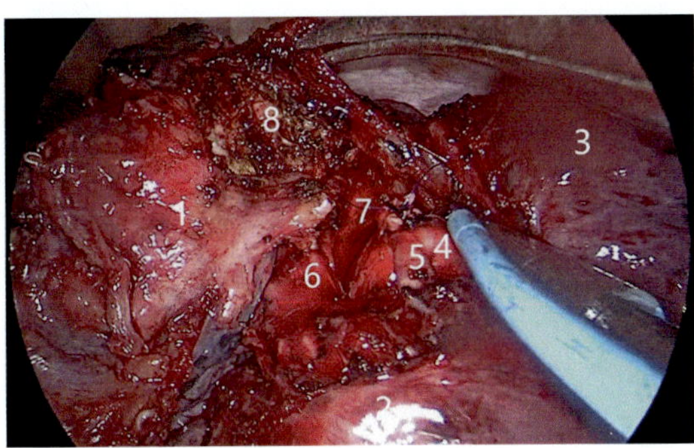

Fig. 6.45 1—Inferior lobe of right lung, 2—middle lobe of right lung, 3—superior lobe of right lung, 4—interlobar trunk of right pulmonary artery, 5—right middle lobe lateral segment artery, 6—right middle lobar bronchus, 7—right middle segment bronchus, 8—right inferior lobar bronchial distal stump. Dissect the lymph node along anterior right middle segment bronchus upward

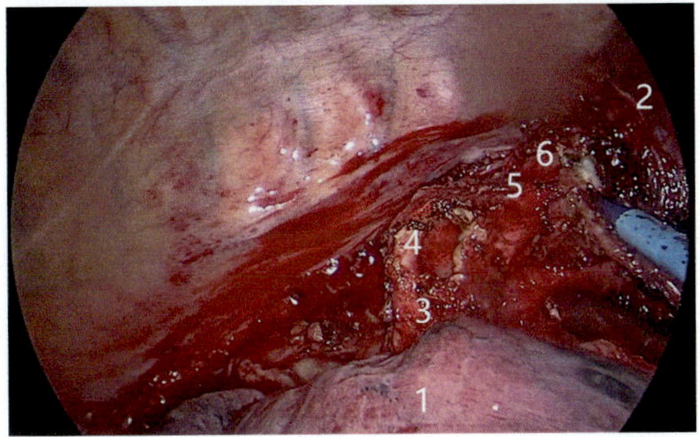

Fig. 6.46 1—Inferior lobe of right lung, 2—superior lobe of right lung, 3—right middle lobar bronchus, 4—right inferior lobar bronchial stump, 5—right middle segment bronchus, 6—right superior lobar bronchus. Dissect the lymph node along anterior right middle segment bronchus upward to anterior right superior lobar bronchus

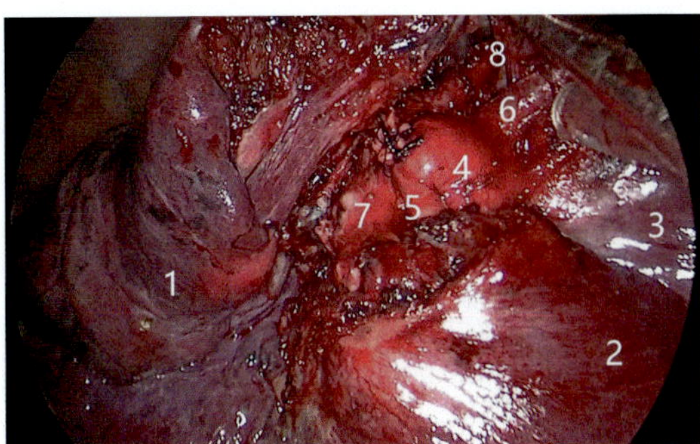

Fig. 6.47 1—Inferior lobe of right lung, 2—middle lobe of right lung, 3—superior lobe of right lung, 4—interlobar trunk of right pulmonary artery, 5—right middle lobe lateral segment artery, 6—posterior segment artery of superior lobe of right lung, 7—right middle lobar bronchus, 8—right superior lobar bronchus. Dissect the lymph node along posterior superior lobe posterior segment artery of right lung upward

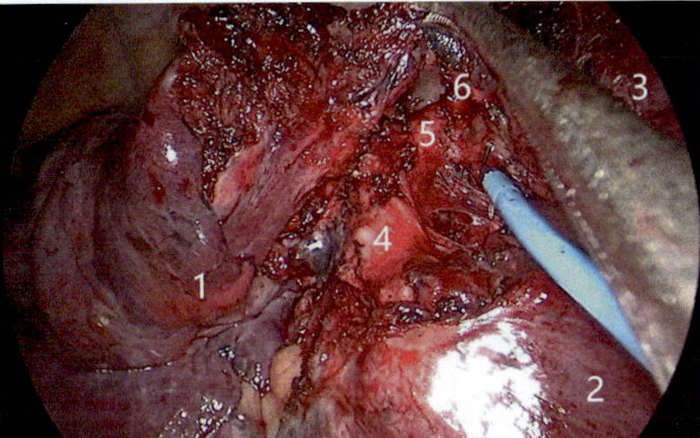

Fig. 6.48 1—Inferior lobe of right lung, 2—middle lobe of right lung, 3—superior lobe of right lung, 4—right middle lobar bronchus, 5—right middle segment bronchus, 6—right superior lobar bronchus. Dissect the lymph node along anterior right superior lobar bronchus upward

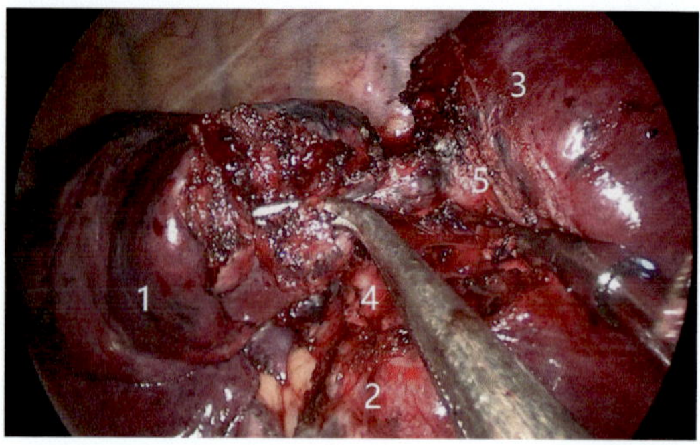

Fig. 6.49 1—Inferior lobe of right lung, 2—middle lobe of right lung, 3—superior lobe of right lung, 4—right middle lobar bronchus, 5—posterior segment bronchus of superior lobe of right lung. Reveal the posterior segment bronchus of superior lobe of right lung and lymph node dissection is finished

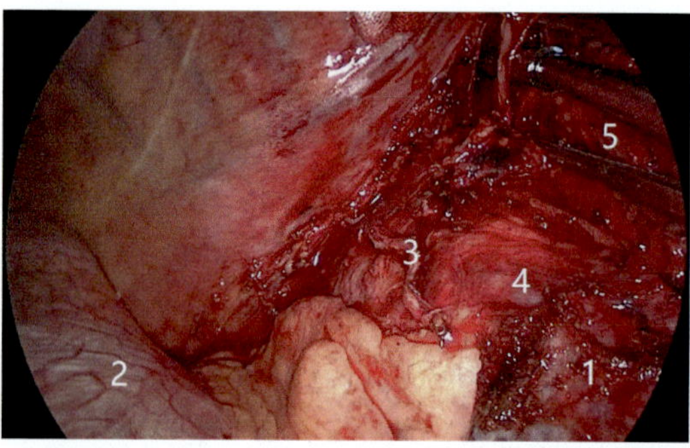

Fig. 6.50 1—Middle lobe of right lung, 2—diaphragm, 3—right inferior pulmonary vein, 4—right middle pulmonary vein, 5—right middle segment bronchus. Dissect the lymph node along posterior right middle segment bronchus upward and reveal right principal bronchus

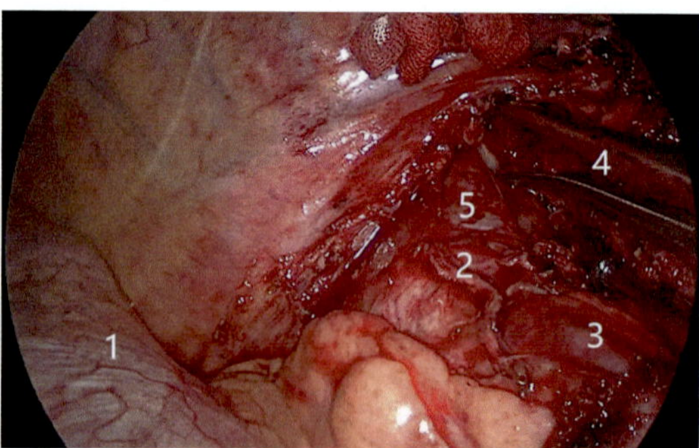

Fig. 6.51 1—Diaphragm, 2—right inferior pulmonary vein, 3—right middle pulmonary vein, 4—right middle segment bronchus, 5—pericardium. Dissect the lymph node along posterior pericardium to anterior esophagus

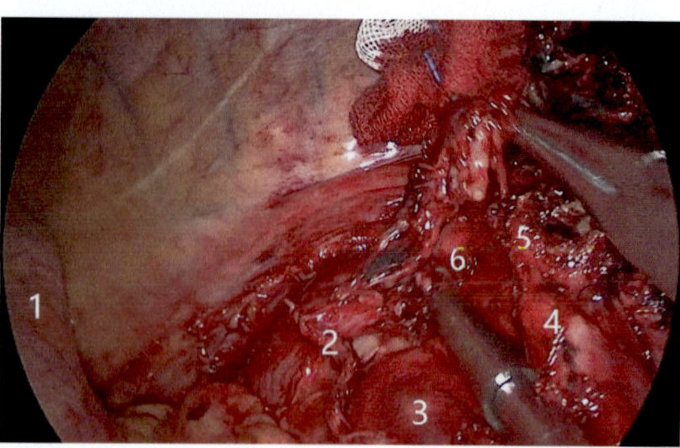

Fig. 6.52 1—Diaphragm, 2—right inferior pulmonary vein stump, 3—right middle pulmonary vein, 4—right middle lobar bronchus, 5—right inferior lobar bronchial stump, 6—left principal bronchus. Reveal left principal bronchus and dissect the lymph node along left principal bronchus downward and backward, and carina lymph node dissection is finished

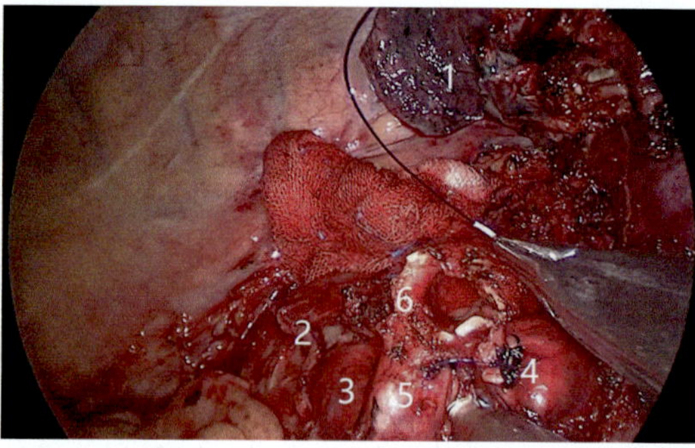

Fig. 6.53 1—Superior lobe of right lung, 2—right inferior pulmonary vein stump, 3—right middle pulmonary vein, 4—interlobar trunk of right pulmonary artery, 5—right middle lobar bronchus, 6—right inferior lobar bronchial stump. Take continuous suture of right inferior lobar bronchial stump

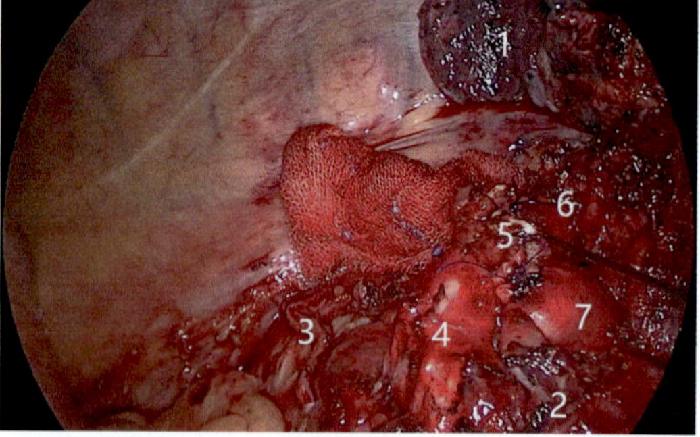

Fig. 6.54 1—Middle lobe of right lung, 2—superior lobe of right lung, 3—right inferior pulmonary vein stump, 4—right middle lobar bronchus, 5—right inferior lobar bronchialstump,6—rightmiddlesegmentbronchus,7—interlobar trunk of right pulmonary artery. Suture is finished

7 Extrapleural Pneumonectomy

Extrapleural Pneumonectomy (EPP) was first reported by Sarot in 1949 for tuberculous empyema. The operation is traumatic and has a high mortality rate. EPP is used in lung cancer mainly in patients with locally advanced or combined malignant hydrothorax, and we also use it for salvage surgery for lung cancer.

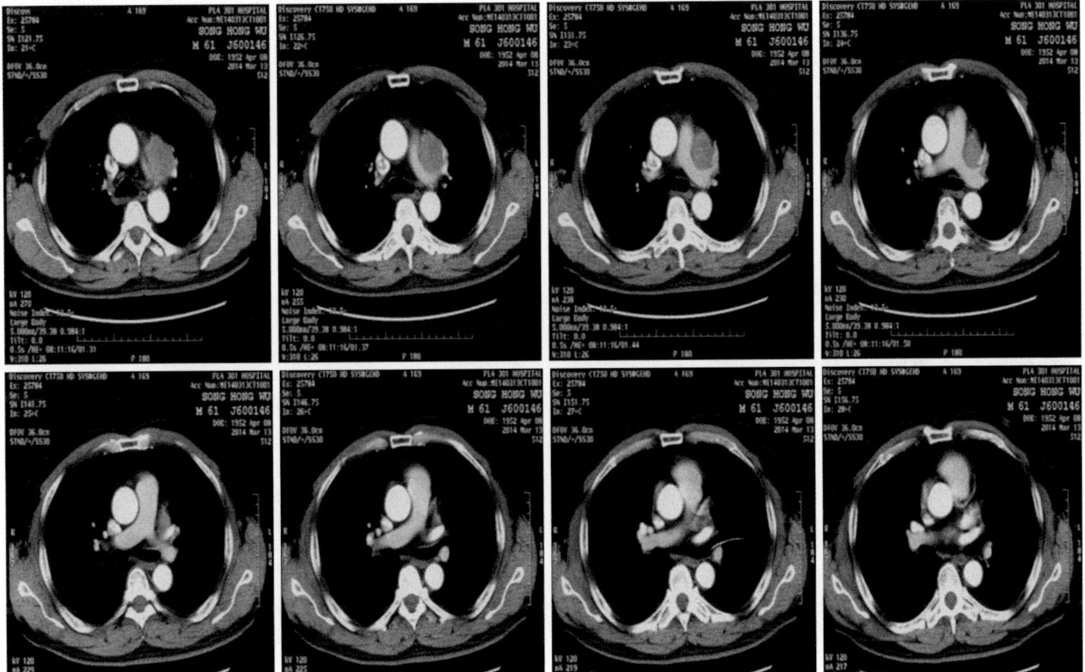

On March 17, 2014, fluoroscopic electronic bronchoscopy + EBUS was performed under general anesthesia and intraoperatively both main, lobar, and segmental lungs and all subsegmental bronchi of the left lung were seen to be patent with no abnormalities.

J. Li, Z. Long, *Atlas of Thoracoscopic Lobectomy with Bronchoplasty*,
https://doi.org/10.1007/978-981-99-5150-5_7

On the same day, a thoracoscopic thoracic exploration was performed under general anesthesia. During the operation, the mass was found to be located above the left pulmonary hilum and behind the phrenic nerve, with a tough texture and poor mobility, a thickened surface pleura, tight adhesions to the left upper lung, pericardium and aorta, and enlarged lymph nodes with a diameter of 0.5–1.0 cm in the pulmonary hilum and interlobular, lymph nodes were tough in texture and grayish black in color. Some tumor tissues and hilar, interlobular and subprotuberant lymph nodes were biopsied after the operation. Postoperative pathology returned low differentiated squamous carcinoma with no metastasis in the lymph nodes.

From March 28, 2014 to May 2, 2014, docetaxel 40 mg + injectable cisplatin 40 mg/week chemotherapy was applied and completed for 6 weeks. IMRT-ARC radiation (40 Gy/200 cGy/20F) for left pulmonary hilum mass was performed from April 1 to April 29. The patient developed elevated transaminases during concurrent chemoradiotherapy, which decreased to normal after hepatoprotective therapy; the lowest white blood cell was 3.98×10^9/L. On May 6, chest enhanced CT showed that the size of left pulmonary hilum tumor was about 3.3 × 2.2 cm. After evaluation, surgical contraindications have been ruled out.

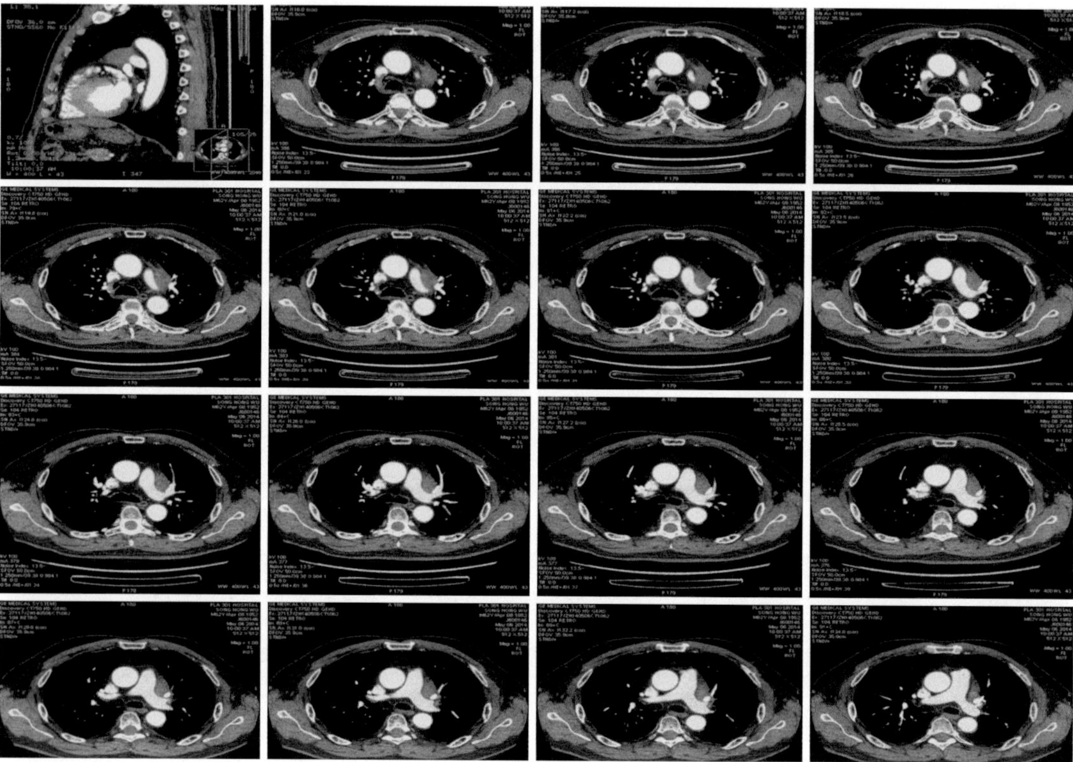

Considering the possibility of pleural dissemination due to intraoperative tumor biopsy, it was decided to perform an EPP with resection of peri-incisional tissue that might cause tumor implantation (Figs. 7.1, 7.2, 7.3, 7.4, 7.5, 7.6, 7.7, 7.8, 7.9, 7.10, 7.11, 7.12, 7.13, 7.14, 7.15, 7.16, 7.17, and 7.18).

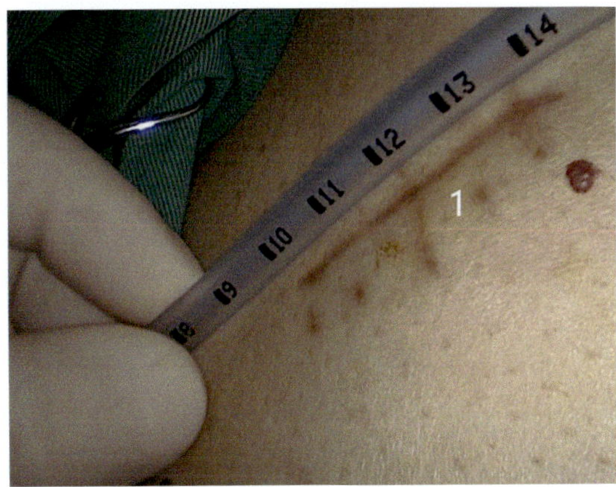

Fig. 7.1 Main operating hole, at anterior fourth intercostal space

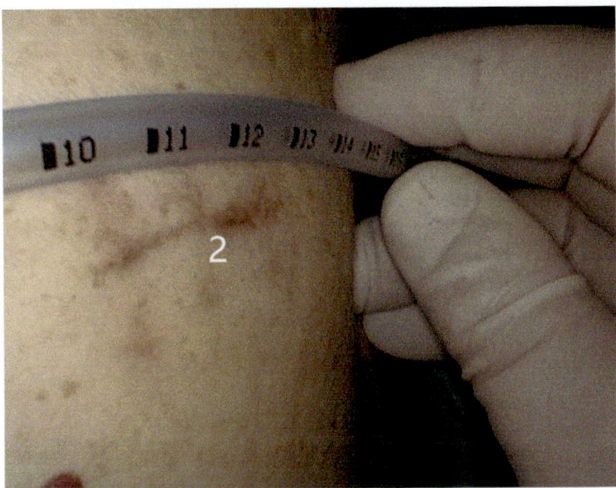

Fig. 7.2 2—Auxiliary operating hole, at sixth intercostal space of posterior axillary line

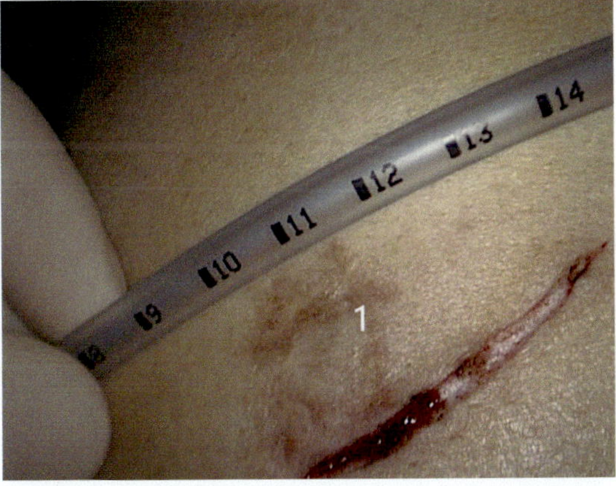

Fig. 7.3 1—Observation hole, at sixth intercostal space of midaxillary line

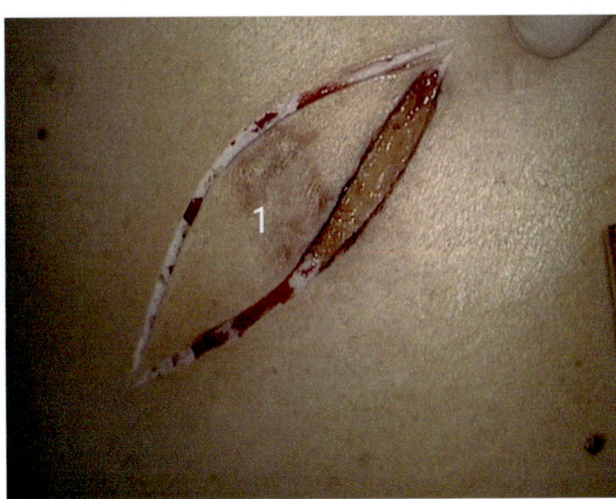

Fig. 7.4 1—Observation hole. Make a fusiform incision and remove the skin around the observation hole

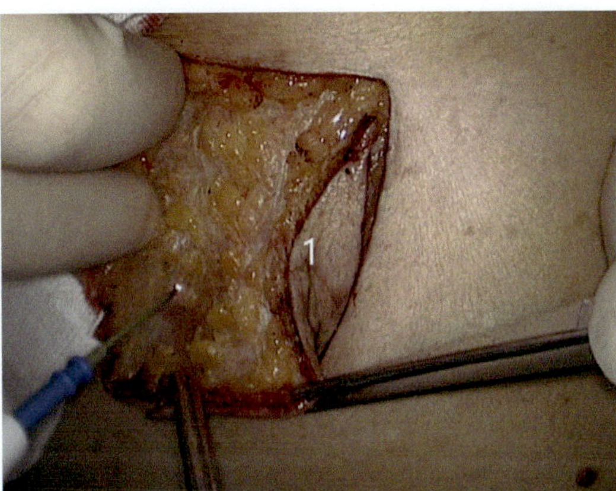

Fig. 7.5 1—Observation hole. Resecting subcutaneous adipose tissue around the observation hole

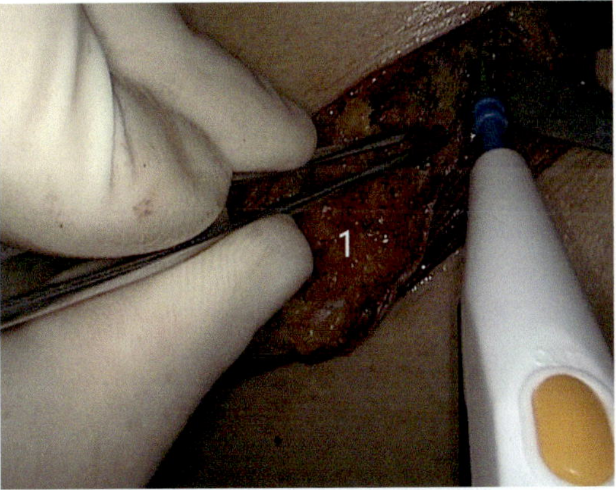

Fig. 7.6 1—Observation hole. Resecting muscle tissue around the incision

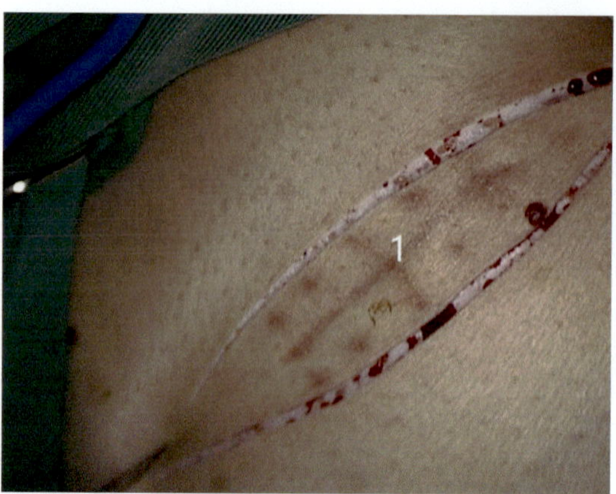

Fig. 7.7 1—Main operating hole. Shuttle-like incision for resecting the skin around main operating hole

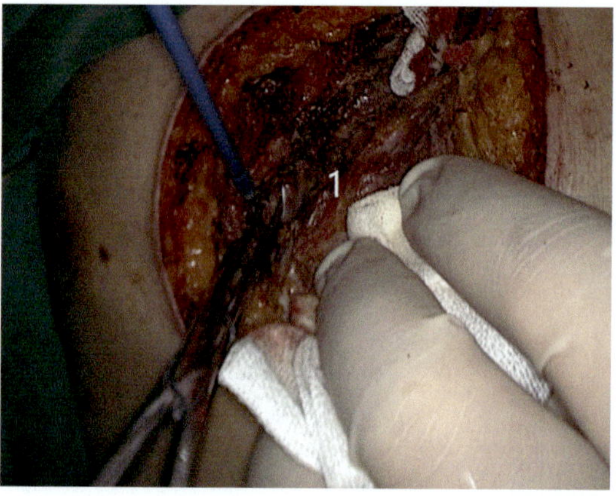

Fig. 7.8 1—Main operating hole. Resecting muscle tissue and adipose tissue around the incision

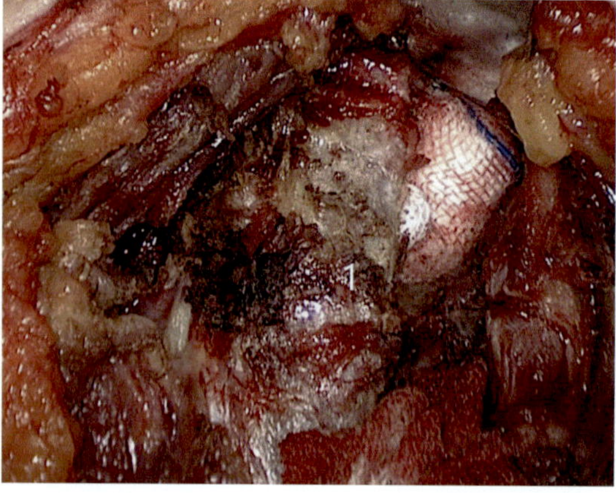

Fig. 7.9 1—Fourth rib. Reveal fourth rib in the area of main operating hole

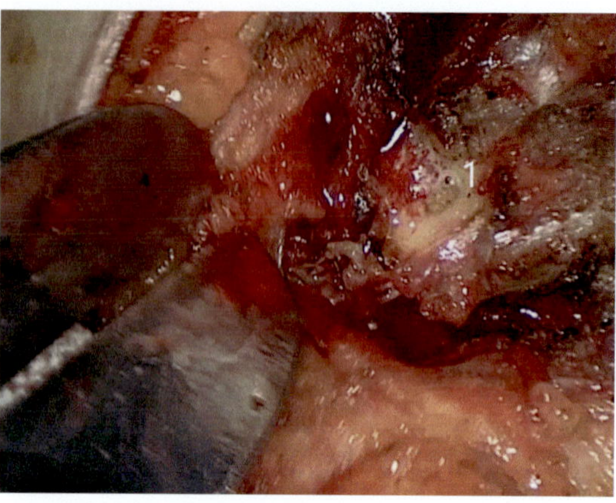

Fig. 7.10 1—Fourth rib. Resect the first part of fourth rib in the area of main operating hole, in order to resect the tumor and make the operation more easily

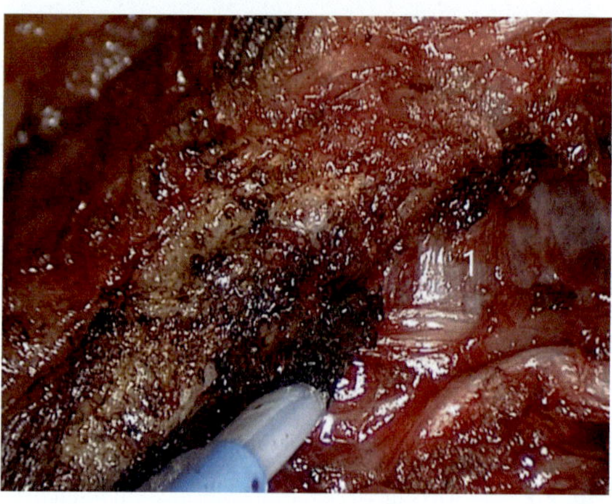

Fig. 7.11 1—Pleura. Dissect outside the pleura along the margin of main operating hole

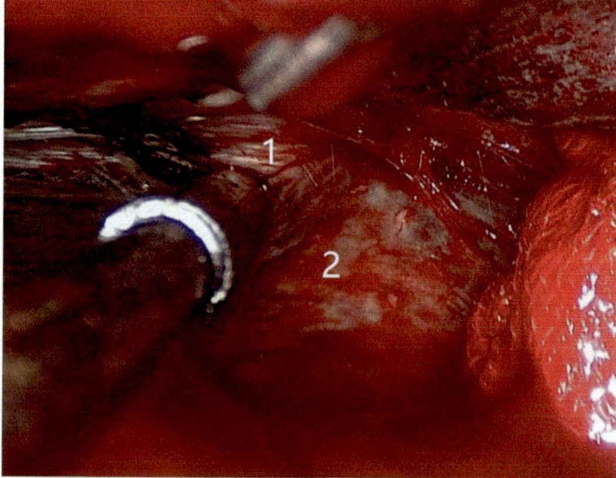

Fig. 7.12 1—Anterior chest wall, 2—pleura. Dissect between anterior chest wall and pleura

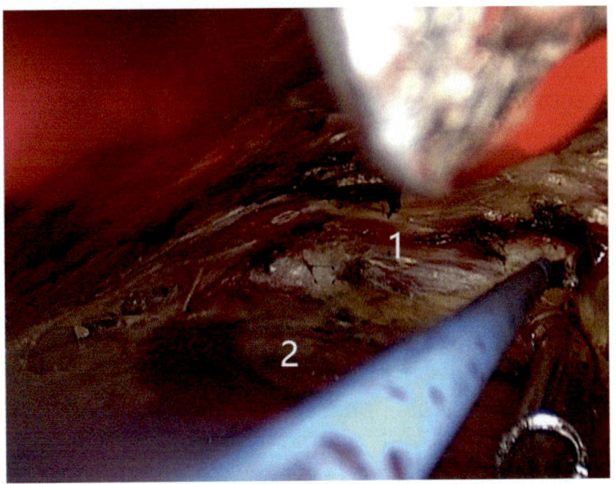

Fig. 7.13 1—Anterior chest wall, 2—pleura. Dissect between anterior chest wall and pleura to the top of thorax

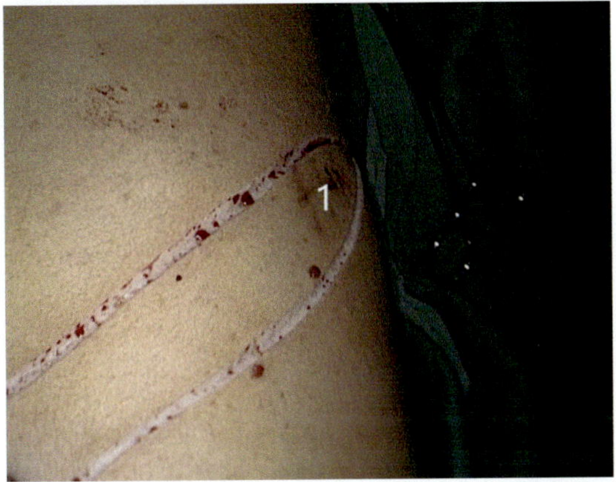

Fig. 7.14 1—Auxiliary operating hole. Take the shuttle-like posterolateral incision forward from auxiliary operating hole

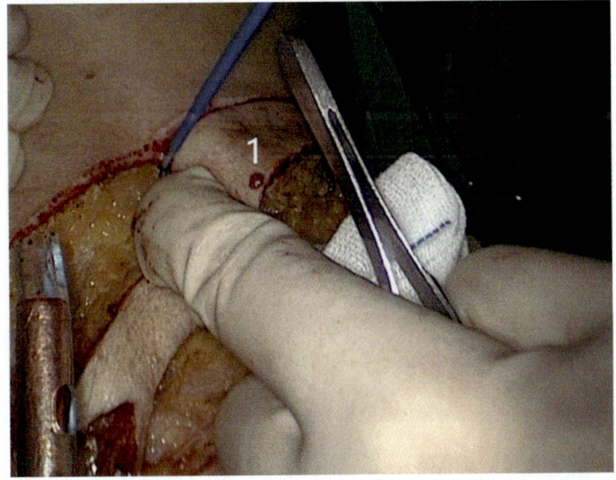

Fig. 7.15 1—Auxiliary operating hole. Resecting muscle tissue and adipose tissue around the auxiliary operating hole

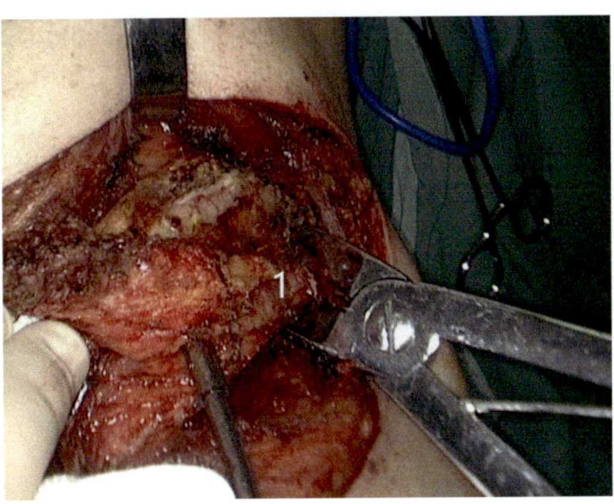

Fig. 7.16 1—Seventh rib. Resect part of seventh rib in the area of auxiliary operating hole

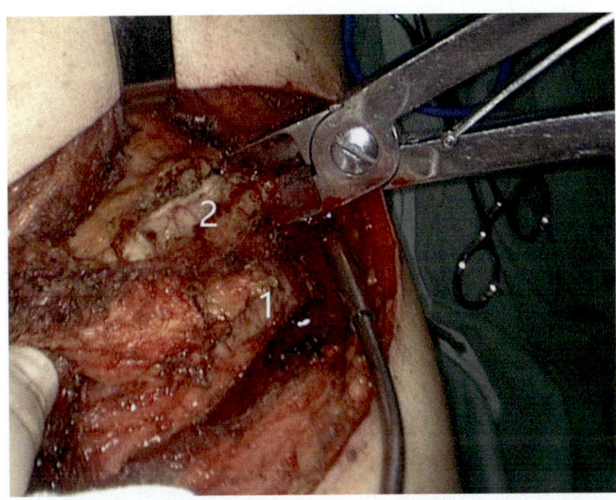

Fig. 7.17 1—Seventh rib, 2 sixth rib. Resect part of sixth rib in the area of auxiliary operating hole

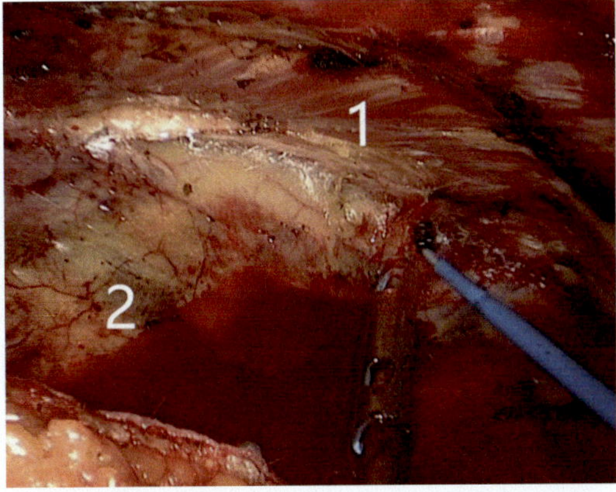

Fig. 7.18 1—Posterior chest wall, 2—pleura. Dissect outside the pleura between posterior chest wall and pleura

The conventional completely pneumonectomy uses a posterolateral incision in the sixth rib from the anterior to the costal cartilage to the posterior to the transverse process. By coincidence, we made a posterolateral incision of more than ten centimeters and completed the entire operation with a thoracoscope after resecting three tissues associated with surgical sites where implantation metastases were likely to occur (Figs. 7.19, 7.20, 7.21, 7.22, 7.23, 7.24, 7.25, 7.26, 7.27, 7.28, 7.29, 7.30, 7.31, 7.32, 7.33, 7.34, 7.35, 7.36, 7.37, 7.38, 7.39, 7.40, 7.41, 7.42, 7.43, 7.44, 7.45, 7.46, 7.47, 7.48, 7.49, 7.50, 7.51, 7.52, 7.53, 7.54, 7.55, 7.56, 7.57, 7.58, 7.59, 7.60, 7.61, 7.62, 7.63, 7.64, 7.65, 7.66, 7.67, 7.68, 7.69, 7.70, 7.71, 7.72, 7.73, 7.74, 7.75, 7.76, and 7.77).

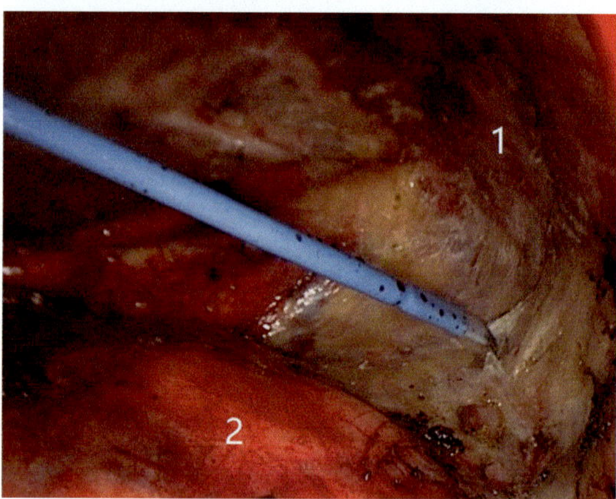

Fig. 7.19 1—Posterior chest wall; 2—pleura. Dissect from posterior chest wall to the top of thorax

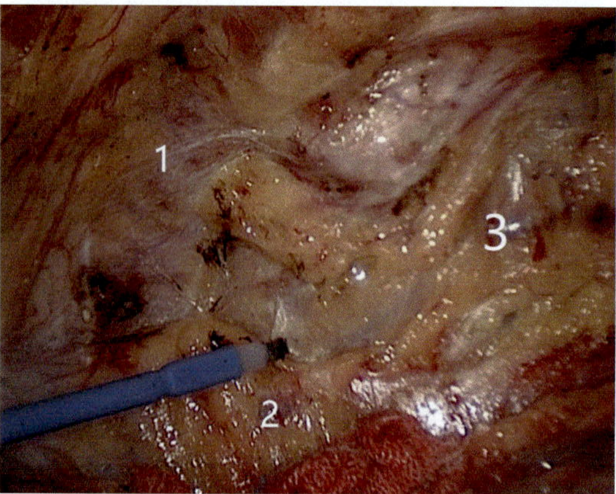

Fig. 7.20 1—Anterior chest wall, 2—pleura, 3—internal thoracic veins. Dissect inward from anterior chest wall

Summary: Extrapleural Pneumonectomy (EPP) is a very radical surgical procedure for thoracic tumors. The whole procedure is located outside the pleural cavity, so that the whole procedure is isolated from the tumor, en-bloc resection, which is radical in the surgical sense; the characteristic of this case is that three surgical exploration incisions were removed for the purpose of radical treatment, thus providing the possibility of thoracoscopic EPP.

In this case, extrapleural separation was performed thoracoscopically from both anterior and posterior directions, achieving the same results as open thoracotomy and providing good material for similar procedures in the future.

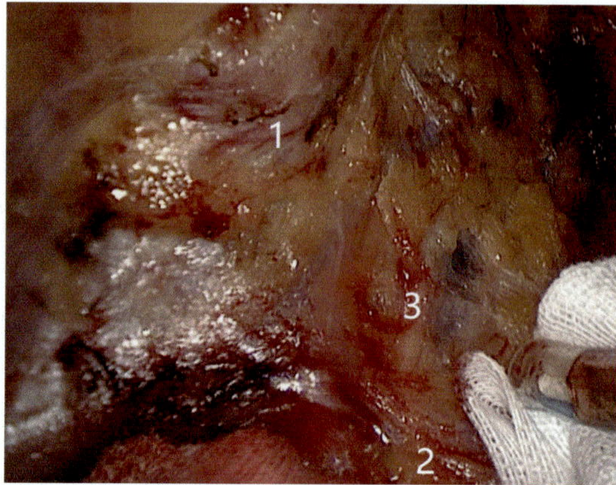

Fig. 7.21 1—Anterior chest wall, 2—pleura, 3—vagus. Dissect and reveal vagus from anterior chest wall inward and upward

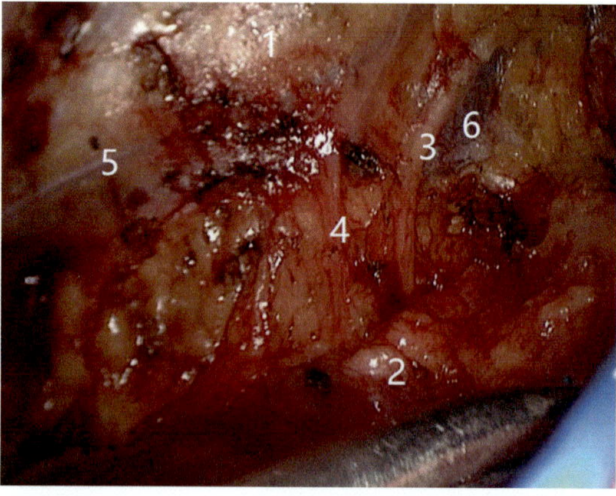

Fig. 7.22 1—Anterior chest wall, 2—pleura, 3—vagus, 4—phrenic nerve, 5—internal thoracic veins, 6—left innominate vein. Continue to dissect inward and upward and reveal phrenic nerve and left innominate vein

In this case, the surgical separation was started from the main operating hole, and the initial extrapleural separation of the anterior and lateral thoracic wall was performed, while the posterior lateral dissociated meeting was performed from the secondary operating hole. The difficulty in the dissociating of the top thoracic region should be noted to distinguish the phrenic nerve from the vagus nerve to prevent accidental injury to the vagus nerve stem, and attention should be paid to protecting the thoracic duct when separating above the aortic arch, and gentle operation and blunt separation should be used to help prevent injury to the thoracic duct; the descending aorta anterior separation should pay attention to the arterial branches emanating from the aorta, accurate hemostasis, and prevent tearing of the root of the vessel. Since the mediastinal pleura has been stripped from the surface of the aorta, aortic vessel suturing has a high degree of difficulty and should be highly attended to.

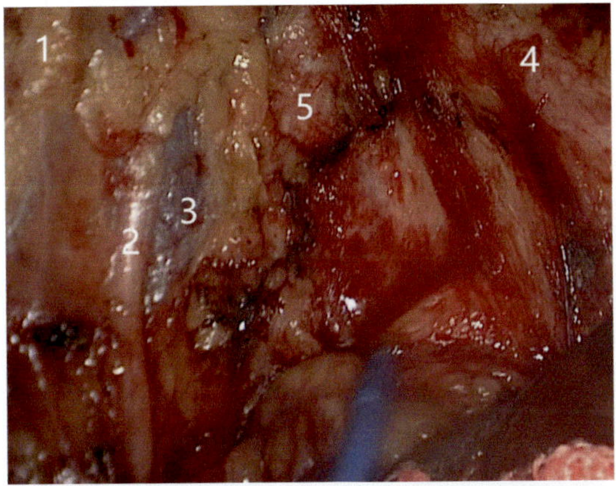

Fig. 7.23 1—Anterior chest wall, 2—vagus, 3—left innominate vein, 4—posterior chest wall, 5—left subclavian artery. Continue to dissect backward and upward to the top of thorax and reveal left subclavian artery

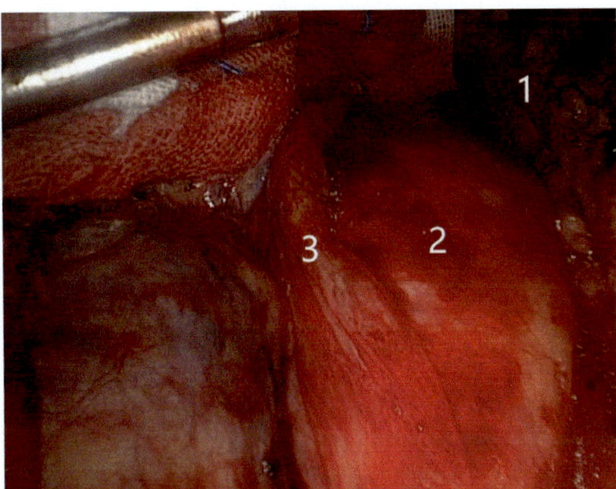

Fig. 7.25 1—Posterior chest wall, 2—descending aorta, 3—pleura. Remove visceral pleura forward on the surface of aorta

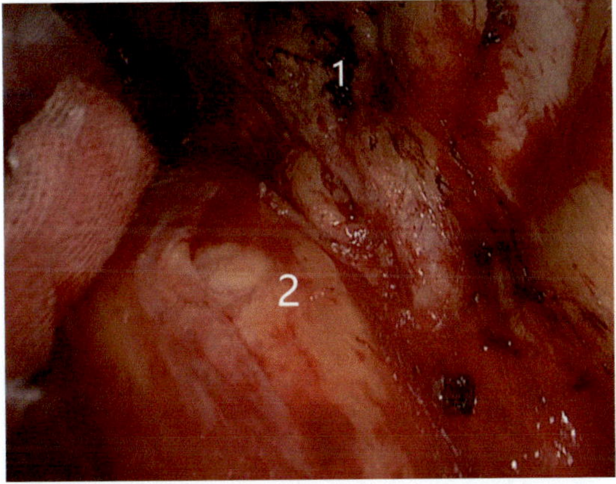

Fig. 7.24 1—Posterior chest wall, 2—descending aorta. Dissect descending aorta inward and forward from posterior chest wall and reveal it, and care should be taken not to damage the thoracic duct when dissecting the aortic arch, which was not shown in this case

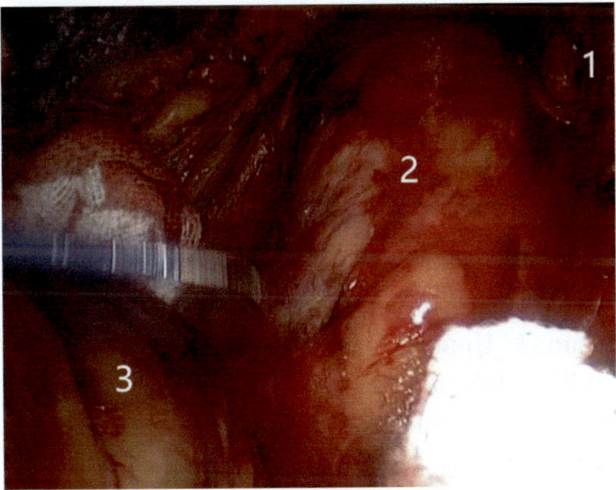

Fig. 7.26 1—Posterior chest wall, 2—descending aorta, 3—pleura. Remove visceral pleura on the surface of aorta completely

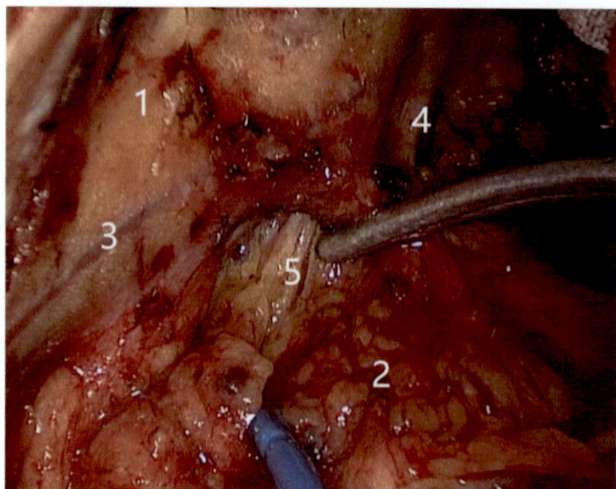

Fig. 7.27 1—Anterior chest wall, 2—pleura, 3—internal thoracic veins, 4—vagus, 5—phrenic nerve. Dissect the phrenic nerve from the top of thorax inward and downward

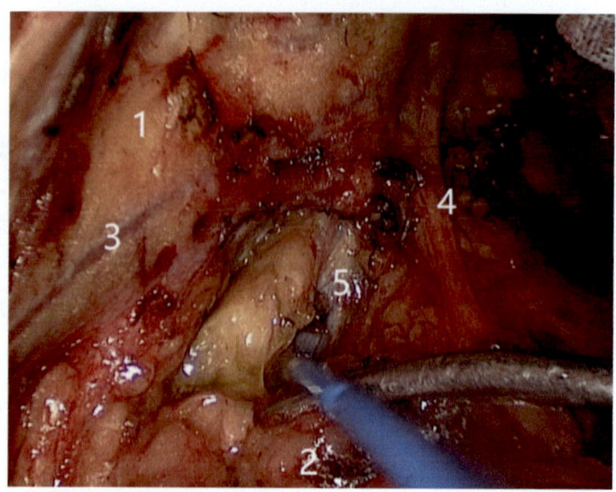

Fig. 7.29 1—Anterior chest wall, 2—pleura, 3—internal thoracic veins, 4—vagus, 5—left innominate vein. Continue to dissect downward and inward along the surface of innominate vein

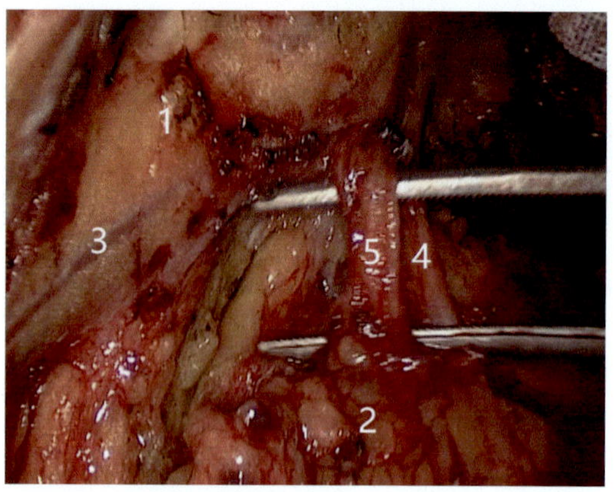

Fig. 7.28 1—Anterior chest wall, 2—pleura, 3—internal thoracic veins, 4—vagus, 5—phrenic nerve. Dissect the phrenic nerve and cut it off

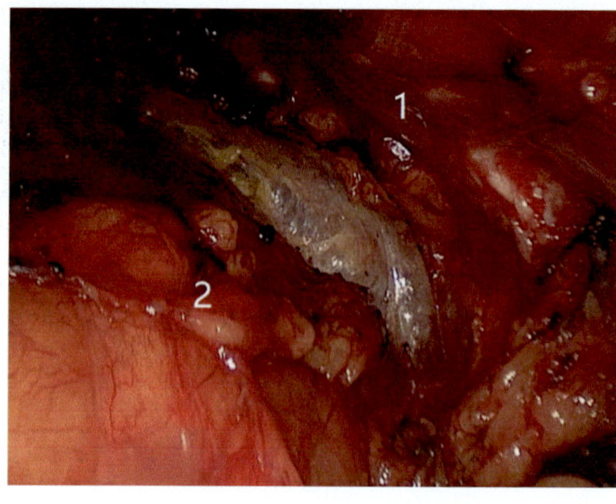

Fig. 7.30 1—Anterior chest wall, 2—pleura and left pericardial fat pad. Dissect downward and inward along anterior chest wall, and dissect pleura and left pericardial fat pad together from the surface of pericardium

The dissection of the lymph nodes of the pulmonary artery window can be found in the Chap. 4 "Upper Lobe of the Left Lung."

The difficulty in resection of the diaphragmatic is in revealing it, the deep location of the diaphragmatic angle makes it difficult to operate, and thoracoscopy is performed with good results with different angles of viewing the operation anteriorly and posteriorly.

Pericardial reconstruction can also be performed using a patch, and in this case, good results were also achieved by using a greater omentum for pericardial reconstruction, and the bronchial stump can also be encapsulated, killing two birds with one stone/attaining two objectives by a single move. However, it should be noted that in emaciated patients, the greater omentum is thin and not suitable for pericardial reconstruction.

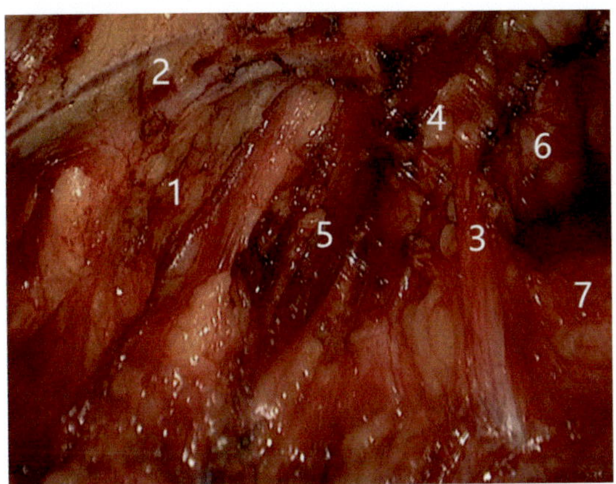

Fig. 7.31 1—Anterior chest wall, 2—internal thoracic veins, 3—vagus, 4—phrenic nerve, 5—left innominate vein, 6—left subclavian artery, 7—aortic arch. Dissect from the top of thorax downward to reveal aortic arch

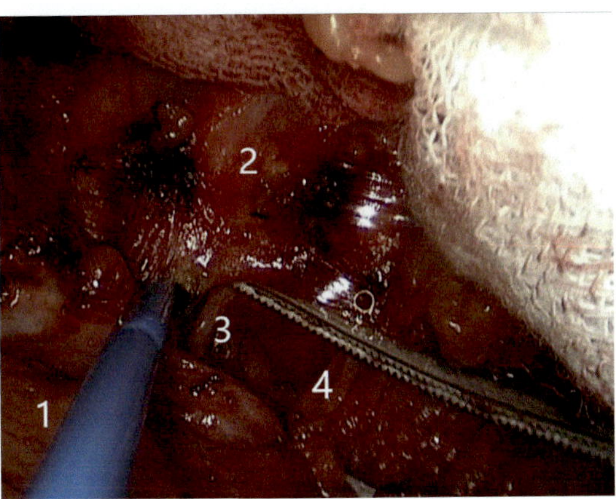

Fig. 7.33 1—Pleura, 2—descending aorta, 3—bronchial artery, 4—bronchial artery. Dissect inward along anterior descending aorta to reveal bronchial artery originating from aorta, and ligature and cut off

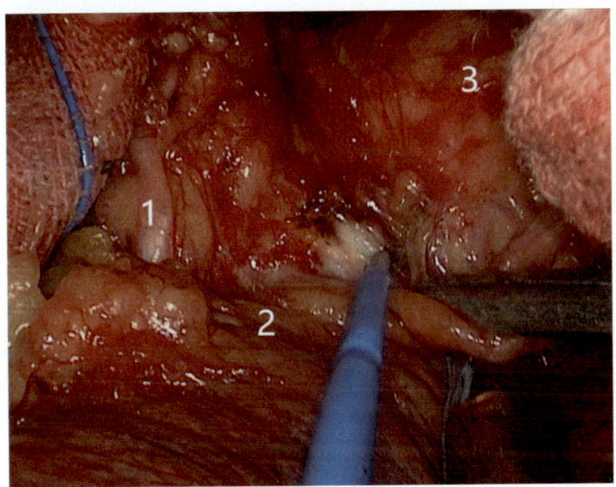

Fig. 7.32 1—Vagus, 2—pleura, 3—aortic arch. Dissect along aortic arch downward

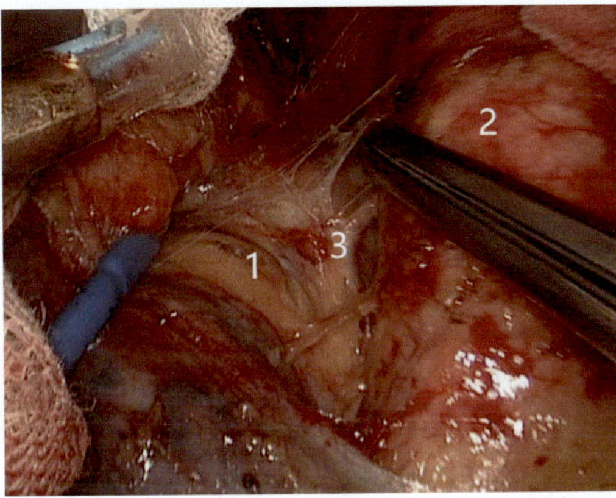

Fig. 7.34 1—Pleura, 2—descending aorta, 3—bronchial artery. Dissect inward and downward along anterior descending aorta, and ligature the branch originating from aorta

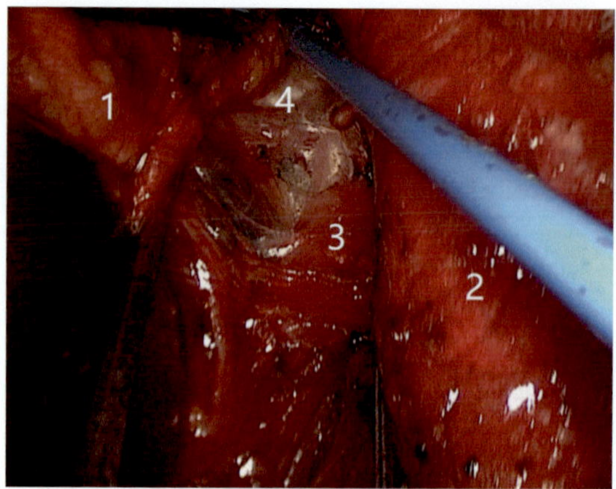

Fig. 7.35 1—Pleura, 2—descending aorta, 3—esophagus, 4—left principal bronchus. Dissect and reveal esophagus and left principal bronchus along anterior descending aorta inward

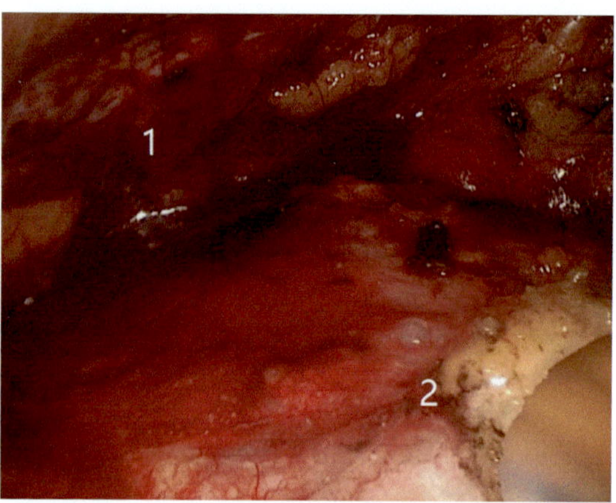

Fig. 7.36 1—Anterior chest wall, 2—pericardium. Cut the pericardium in front of phrenic nerve

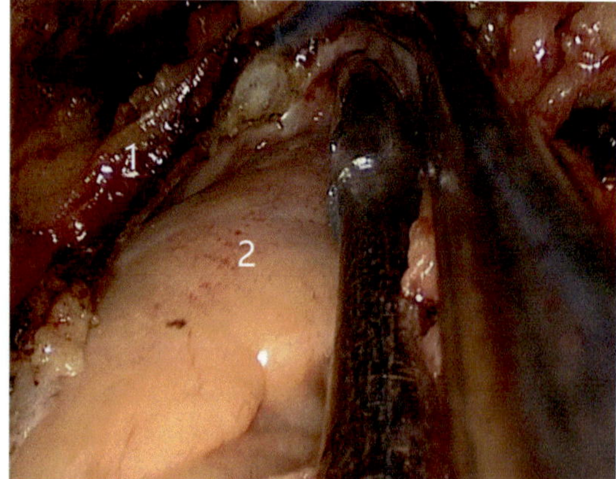

Fig. 7.37 1—Pericardium, 2—left ventricle. Continue to open the pericardium and open pericardial reflection

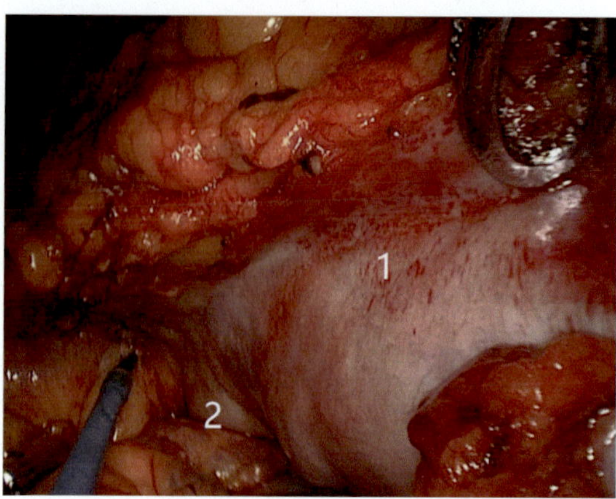

Fig. 7.38 1—Pericardium, 2—superior pulmonary vein. Pull the pericardium backward and reveal left superior pulmonary vein

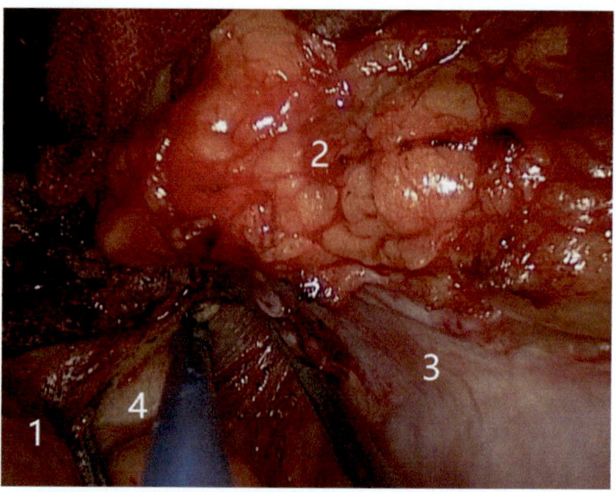

Fig. 7.39 1—Left ventricle, 2—pleura, 3—pericardium, 4—left pulmonary artery. Open the adventitia of anterior left pulmonary artery

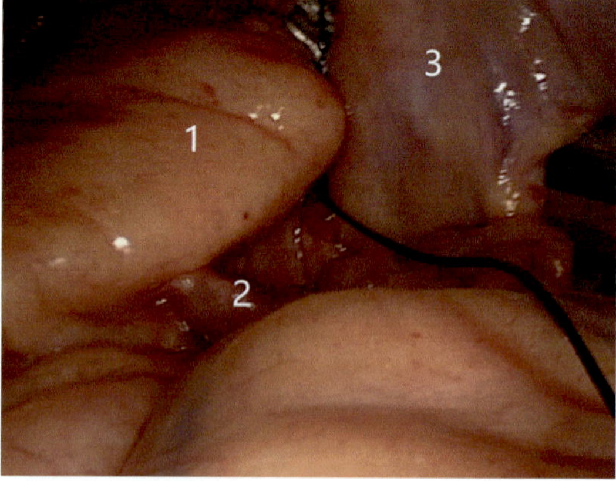

Fig. 7.40 1—Left ventricle, 2—left auricle, 3—superior pulmonary vein. Overlap line of left superior pulmonary vein and pull

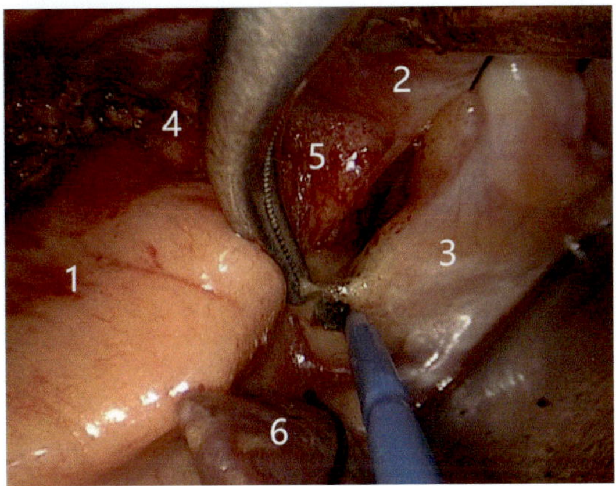

Fig. 7.41 1—Left ventricle, 2—pericardium, 3—superior pulmonary vein aorta, 4—aortic arch, 5—left pulmonary artery, 6—left auricle. Open the pericardial reflection between superior pulmonary vein and left pulmonary artery, dissect inferior pulmonary artery

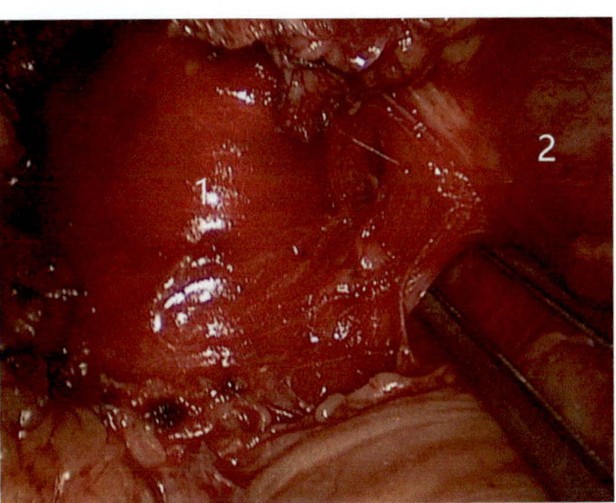

Fig. 7.43 1—Ascending aorta, 2—left pulmonary artery. Open the pericardial reflection between aorta and pulmonary artery, dissect superior left pulmonary artery completely

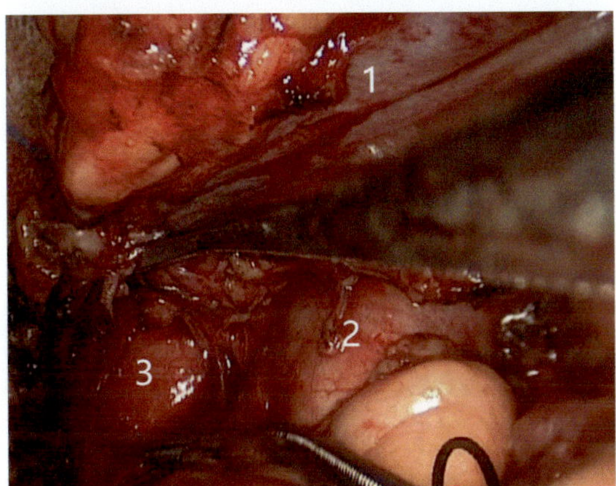

Fig. 7.42 1—Pericardium, 2—left pulmonary artery, 3—ascending aorta. Dissect superior pulmonary artery to reveal ascending aorta

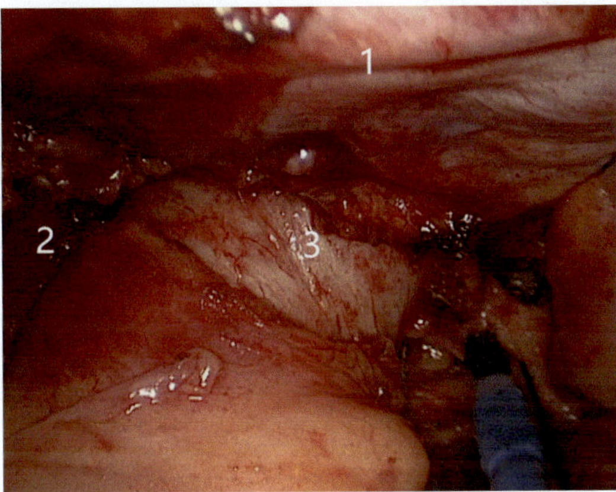

Fig. 7.44 1—Pericardium, 2—ascending aorta, 3—left pulmonary artery. Dissect posterior left pulmonary artery

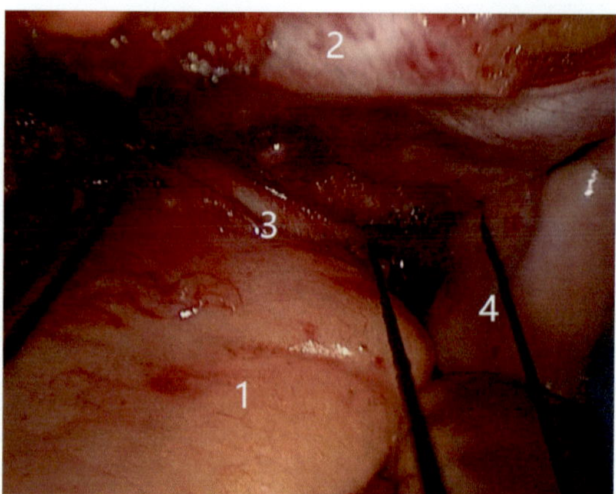

Fig. 7.45 1—Left ventricle, 2—pericardium, 3—left pulmonary artery, 4—superior pulmonary vein. Overlapping line of left pulmonary artery

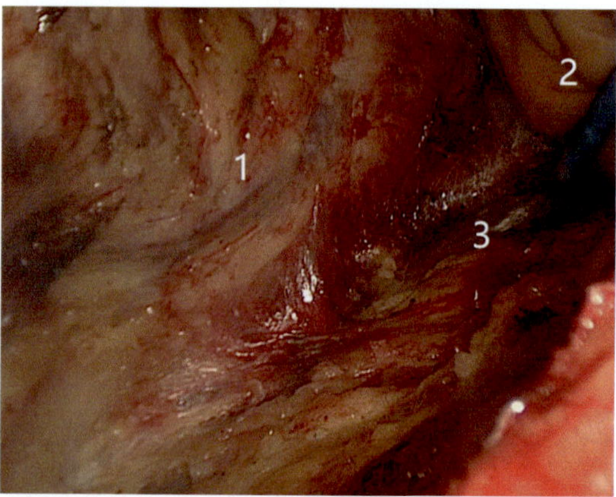

Fig. 7.46 1—Posterior chest wall, 2—pleura, 3—diaphragm. Dissect along posterior chest wall inward and downward, resect visceral pleura on the surface of diaphragm and reveal diaphragms

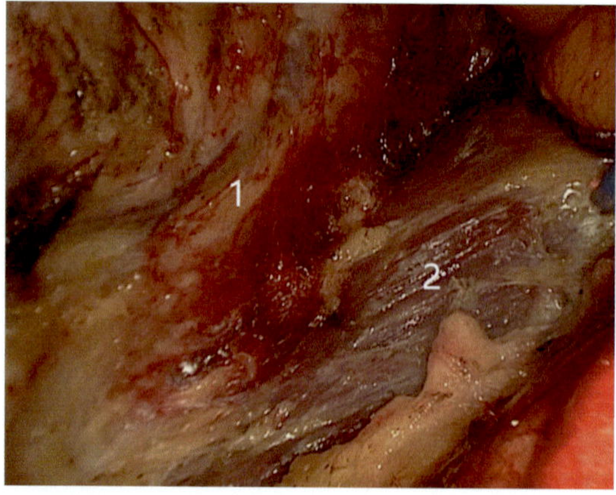

Fig. 7.47 1—Posterior chest wall, 2—diaphragm. Dissect visceral pleura along the surface of diaphragm

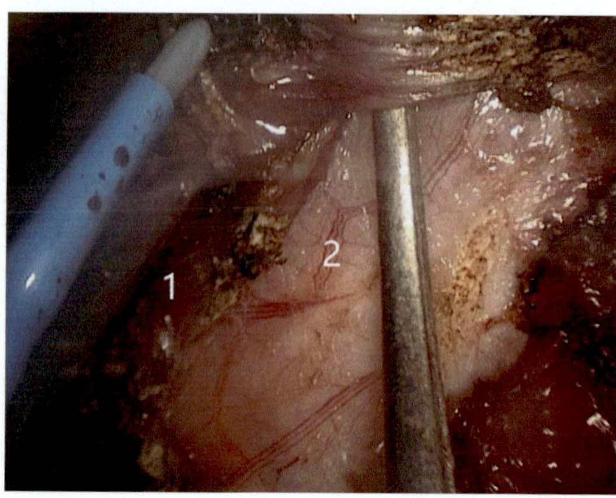

Fig. 7.48 1—Diaphragm, 2—peritoneum. Reveal peritoneum and cut off diaphragm at 2 cm from where the diaphragm attaches to the chest wall

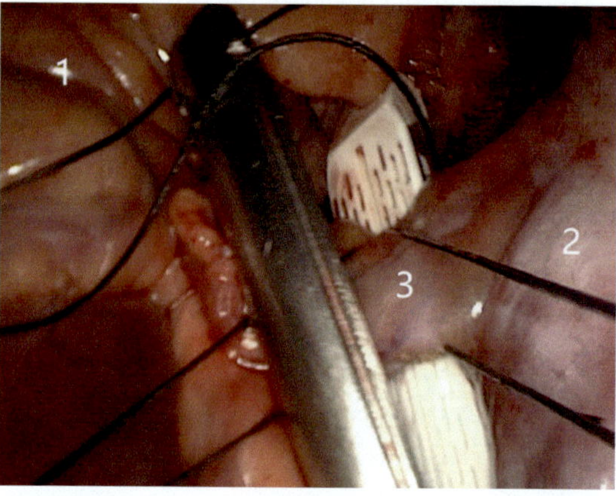

Fig. 7.49 1—Left ventricle, 2—pericardium, 3—superior pulmonary vein. Interrupt superior pulmonary vein with GIA

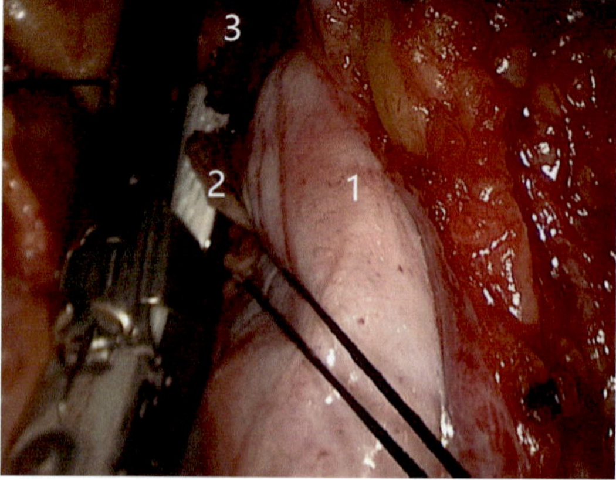

Fig. 7.50 1—Pericardium, 2—superior pulmonary vein stump, 3—left pulmonary artery. Interrupt left pulmonary artery with GIA

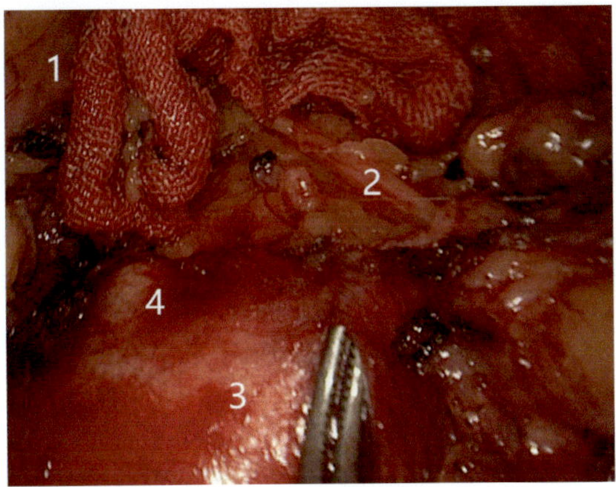

Fig. 7.51 1—Anterior chest wall, 2—vagus, 3—ascending aorta, 4—right brachiocephalic trunk. Dissect along ascending aorta upward and backward

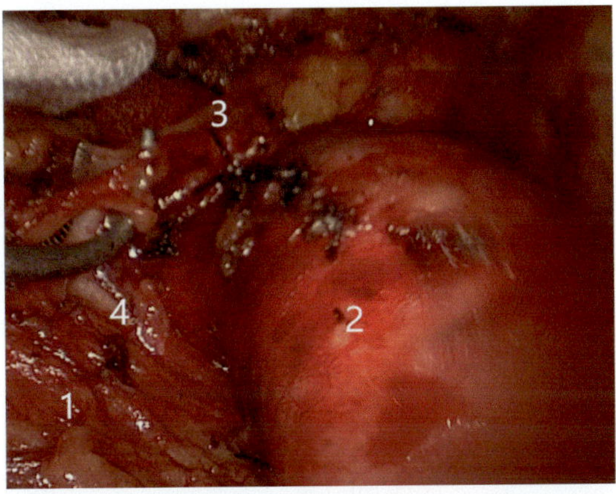

Fig. 7.52 1—Pleura, 2—descending aorta, 3—vagus, 4—left recurrent laryngeal nerve. Dissect vagus to reveal recurrent laryngeal nerve

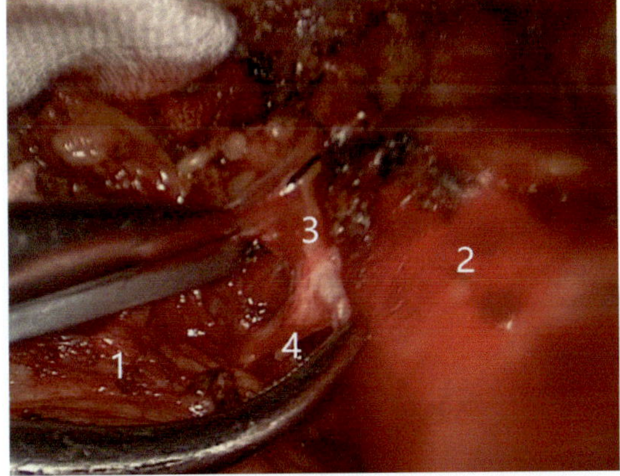

Fig. 7.53 1—Pericardium, 2—descending aorta, 3—vagus, 4—recurrent laryngeal nerve. Dissect vagus

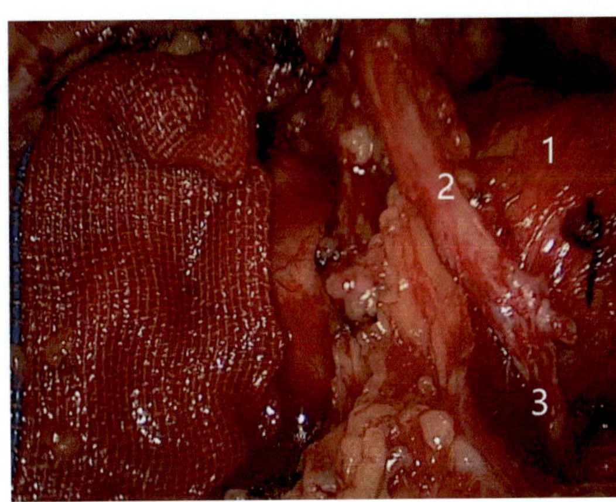

Fig. 7.54 1—Aortic arch, 2—vagus, 3—recurrent laryngeal nerve. Cut off vagus below where the recurrent laryngeal nerve originates from, and recurrent laryngeal nerve reflects behind the aortic arch

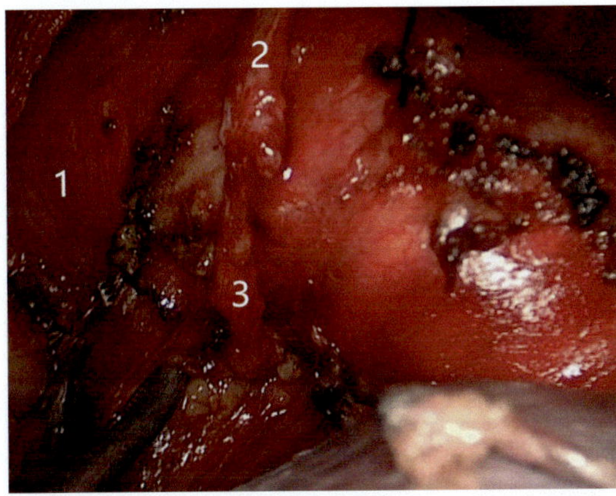

Fig. 7.55 1—Aortic arch, 2—vagus, 3—recurrent laryngeal nerve. Dissect the lymph node near recurrent laryngeal nerve below the aortic arch

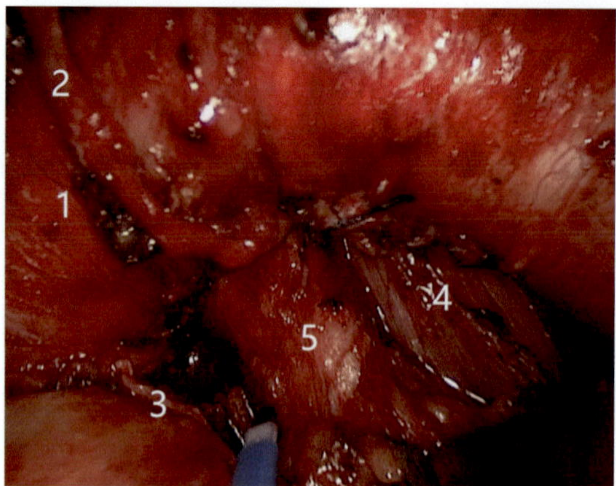

Fig. 7.56 1—Aortic arch, 2—vagus, 3—pulmonary artery stump, 4—esophagus, 5—trachea. Showing the esophagus and trachea after finishing the lymph node dissection

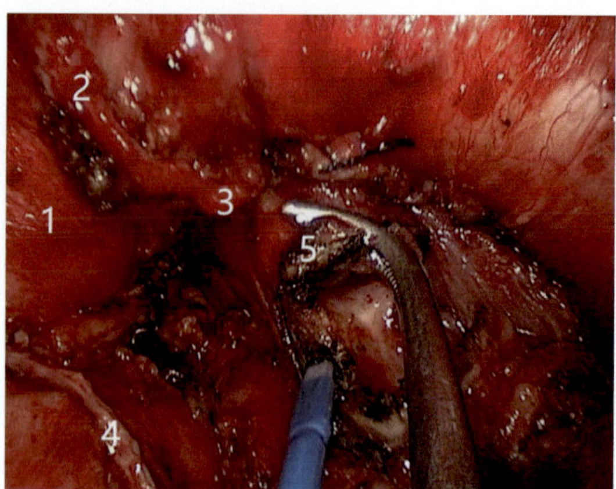

Fig. 7.58 1—Aortic arch, 2—vagus, 3—recurrent laryngeal nerve, 4—pulmonary artery stump, 5—left principal bronchus opening. Cut off left principal bronchus at left principal bronchus opening

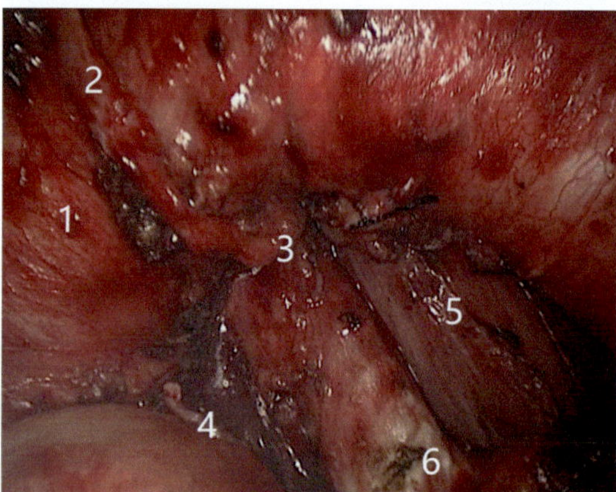

Fig. 7.57 1—Aortic arch, 2—vagus, 3—recurrent laryngeal nerve, 4—pulmonary artery stump, 5—esophagus, 6—left principal bronchus broken end. Cut at left principal bronchus opening

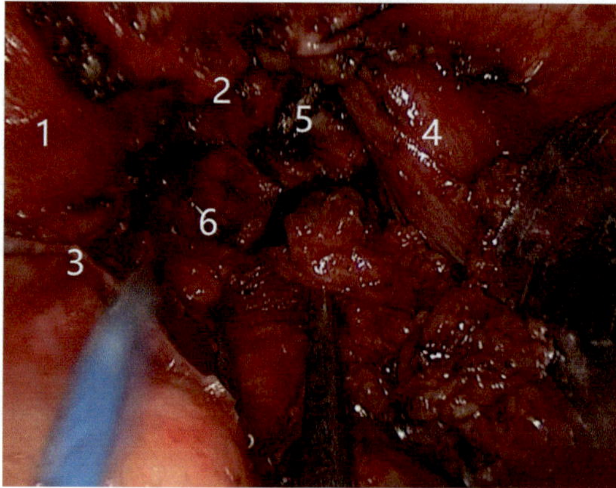

Fig. 7.59 1—Aortic arch, 2—recurrent laryngeal nerve, 3—pulmonary artery stump, 4—esophagus, 5—left principal bronchus opening, 6—right principal bronchus. Dissect the lymph node along right principal bronchus

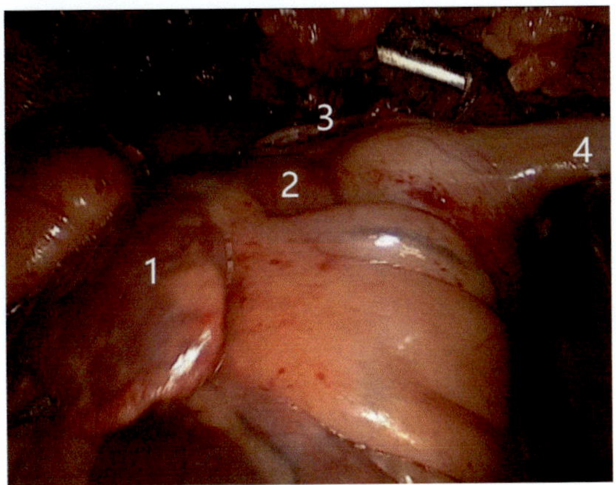

Fig. 7.60 1—Left auricle, 2—left atrium, 3—superior pulmonary vein stump, 4—inferior pulmonary vein. Dissect inferior pulmonary vein and cut it off with GIA

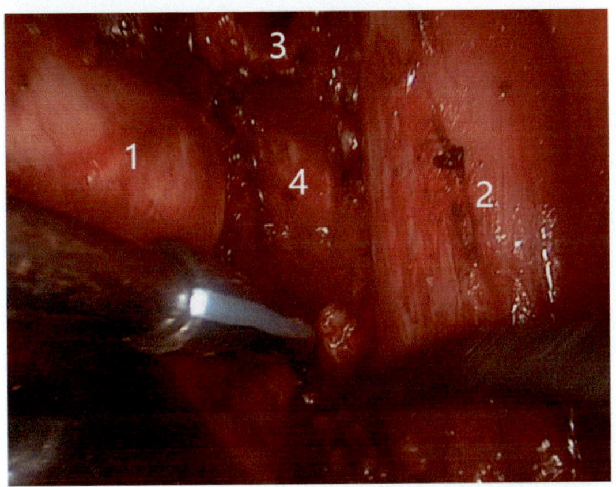

Fig. 7.61 1—Pleura, 2—esophagus, 3—left principal bronchus opening, 4—right principal bronchus. Dissect the lymph node along right principal bronchus downward to the end of right middle segment bronchus

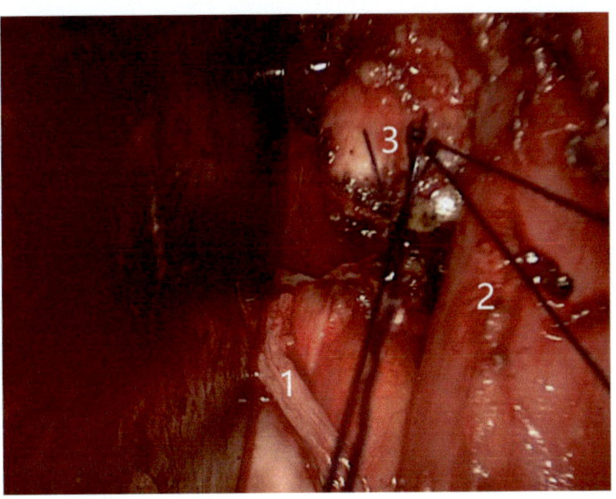

Fig. 7.62 1—Inferior pulmonary vein stump, 2—esophagus, 3—left principal bronchial stump. Suture left principal bronchial stump

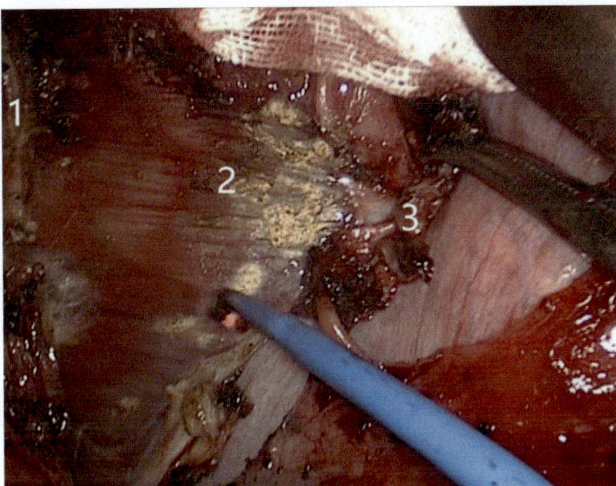

Fig. 7.63 1—Posterior chest wall where the diaphragm attaches, 2—diaphragm, 3—visceral pleura. Cut diaphragm at 2 cm from where the diaphragm attaches

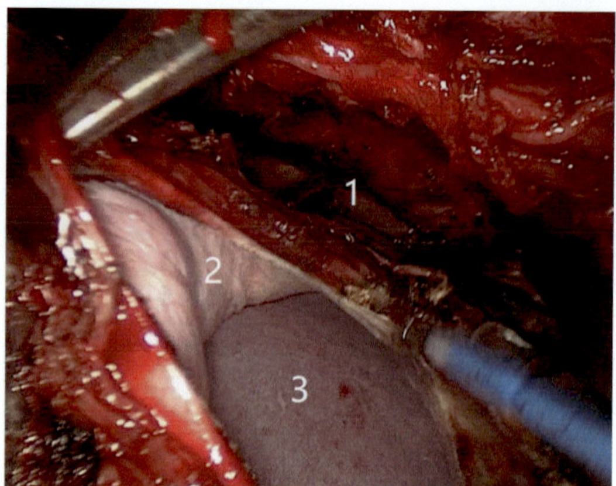

Fig. 7.64 1—Posterior chest wall, 2—diaphragm, 3—spleen. Cut diaphragm circularly at 2 cm from where the diaphragm attaches

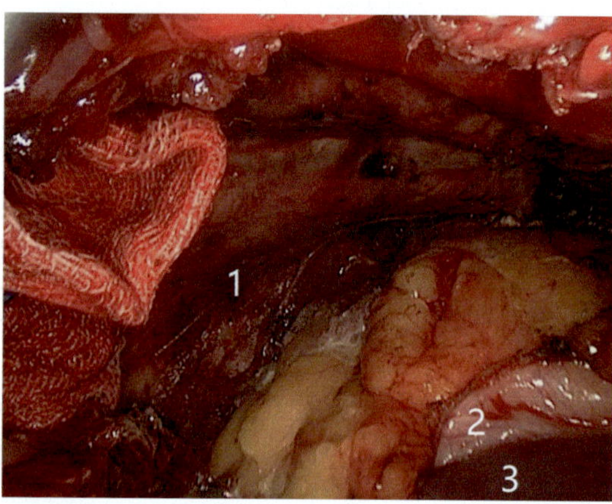

Fig. 7.65 1—Anterior chest wall, 2—diaphragm, 3—spleen. Cut diaphragm circularly at 2cm from where the diaphragm attaches

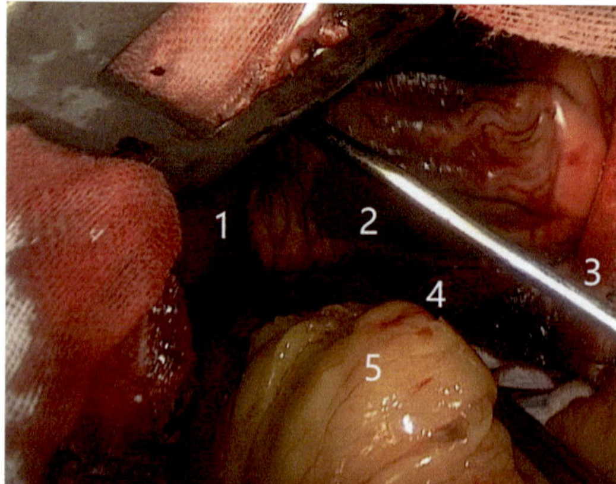

Fig. 7.66 1—Anterior chest wall, 2—heart, 3—descending aorta, 4—diaphragm, 5—greater omentum. Showing diaphragm stump after circular resection of diaphragm

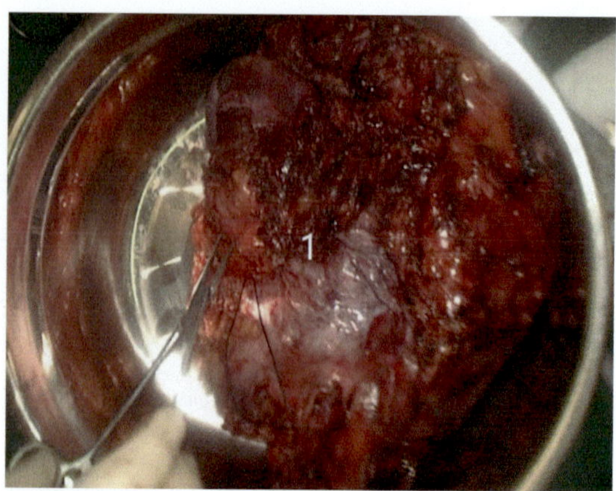

Fig. 7.67 1—Specimen. Take out specimen

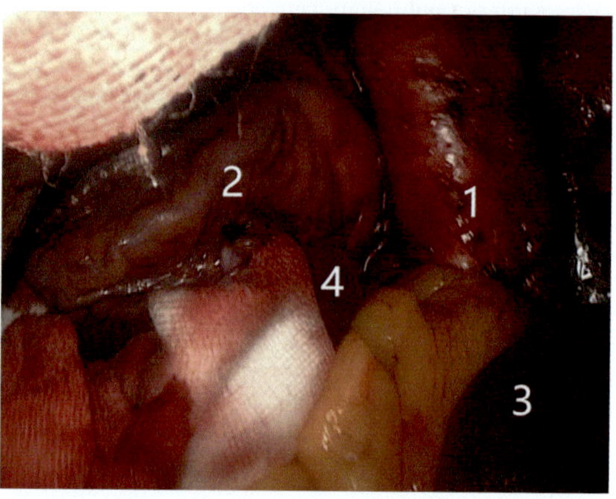

Fig. 7.68 1—Descending aorta, 2—left ventricle, 3—spleen, 4—liver. After resection of diaphragm

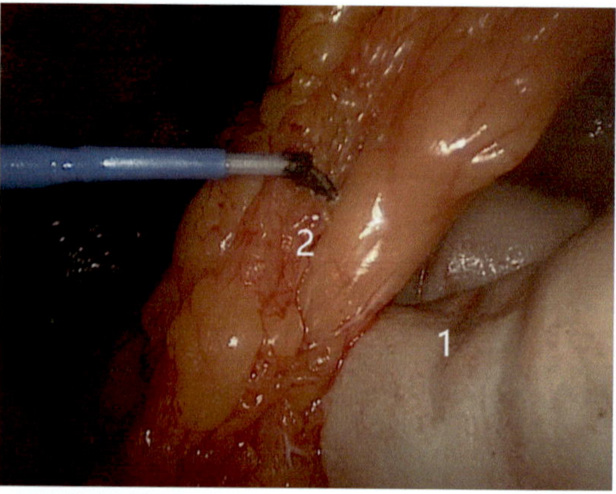

Fig. 7.69 1—Stomach, 2—greater omentum. Dissecting greater omentum

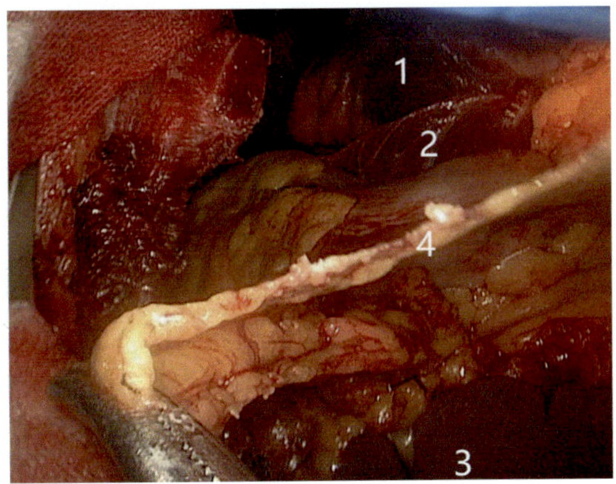

Fig. 7.70 1—Left ventricle, 2—spleen, 3—liver, 4—greater omentum. Dissecting greater omentum

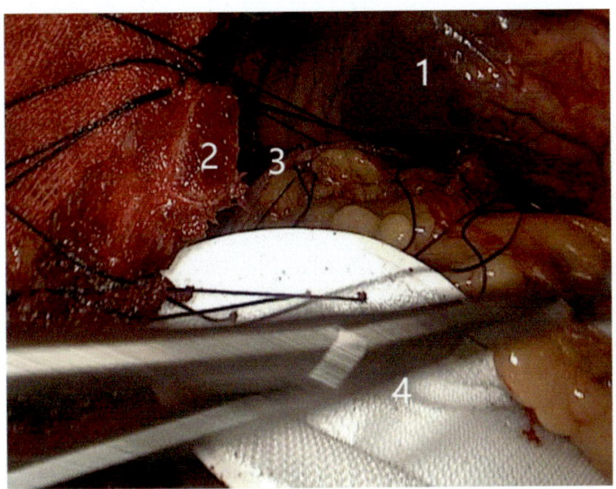

Fig. 7.71 1—Left ventricle, 2—broken end of rib, 3—diaphragm, 4—Bard mesh. Use Bard mesh to reconstruct diaphragm and suture Bard mesh and anterior diaphragm stump

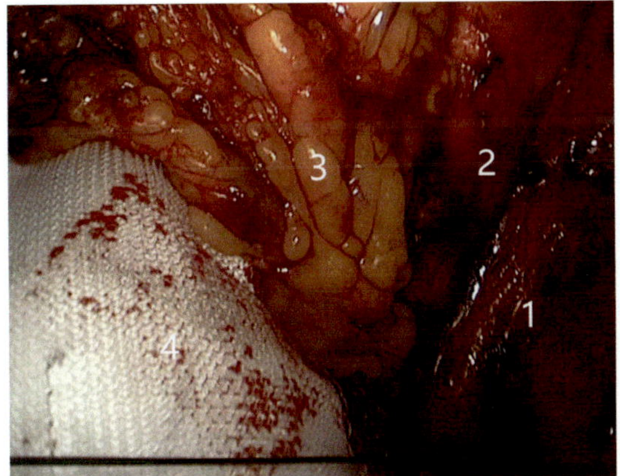

Fig. 7.72 1—Posterior chest wall, 2—descending aorta, 3—greater omentum, 4—Bard mesh

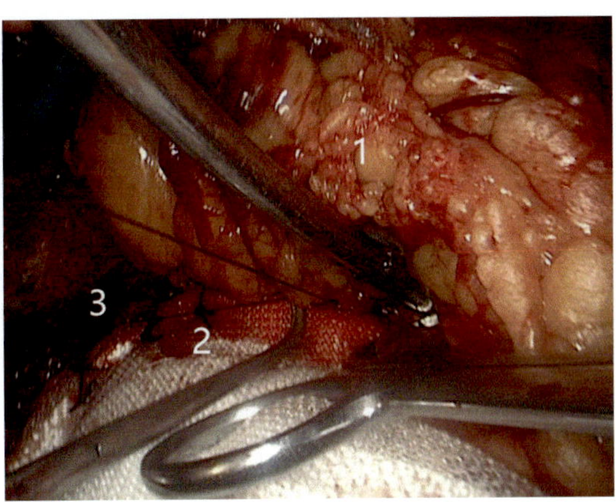

Fig. 7.73 1—Greater omentum, 2—Bard mesh, 3—anterior chest wall. Pull the greater omentum from esophageal hiatus to thoracic cavity

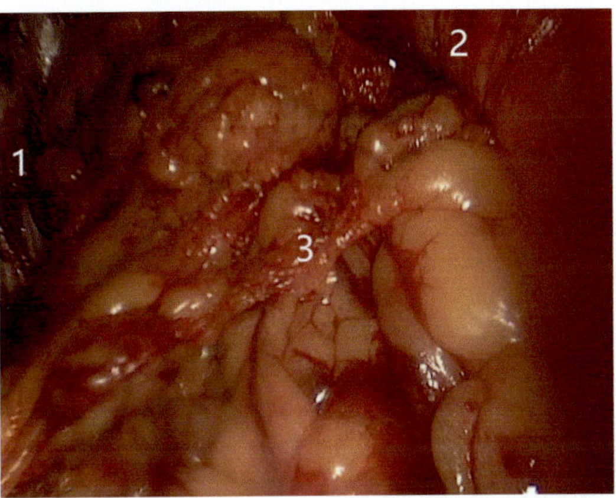

Fig. 7.74 1—Anterior chest wall, 2—descending aorta, 3—greater omentum. Reconstruct pericardium with the greater omentum to cover the left of the heart

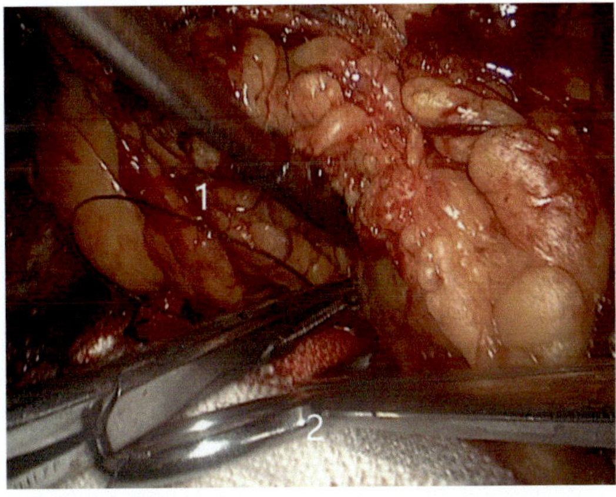

Fig. 7.75 1—Greater omentum, 2—Bard mesh. Suture Bard mesh and greater omentum

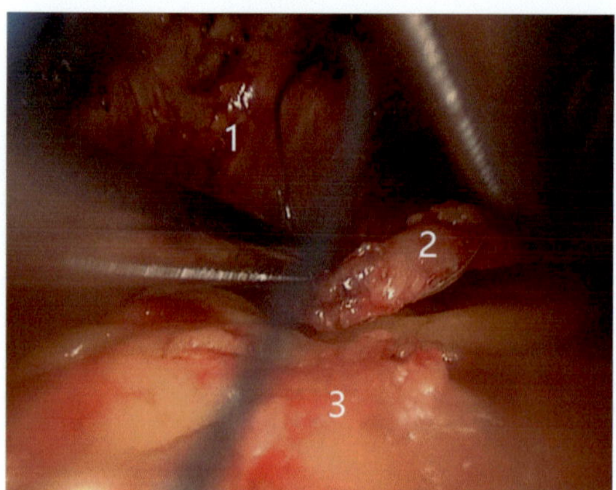

Fig. 7.76 1—Anterior chest wall, 2—pericardium stump, 3—greater omentum. Suture anterior pericardium stump and greater omentum

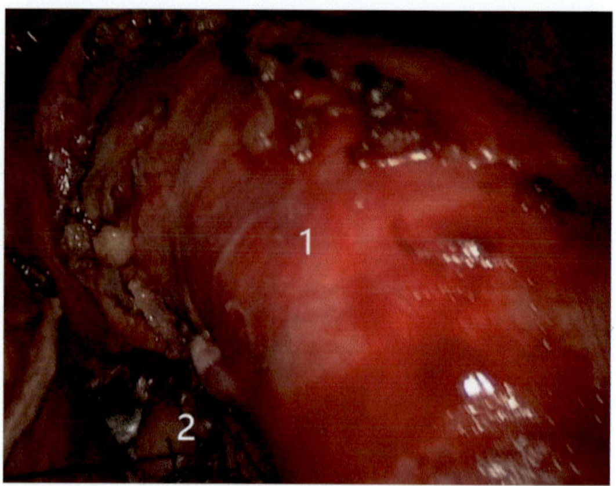

Fig. 7.77 1—Descending aorta, 2—left principal bronchial stump. Suture left principal bronchial stump and greater omentum and embed the stump

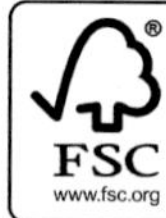

MIX
Papier aus verantwortungsvollen Quellen
Paper from responsible sources
FSC® C105338

If you have any concerns about our products,
you can contact us on
ProductSafety@springernature.com

In case Publisher is established outside the EU,
the EU authorized representative is:
Springer Nature Customer Service Center GmbH
Europaplatz 3, 69115 Heidelberg, Germany

Printed by Libri Plureos GmbH
in Hamburg, Germany